PALEO DIET
THE 4 WEEKS CHALLENGE 30 DAYS PALEO MEAL PLAN

PREFACE

Emma Vickens is a professional nutritionist who has been in the field for years. She completely understands the different types of diet available and which ones are the best for you.

After years of suffering from a digestive disorder and not finding an effective solution, Emma decided to end her suffering by researching the different types of diets and nutritional options available. Years of extensive research resulted in Emma to perfectly understanding the secret of a healthy body and mind. Now she has decided to share this with all her loyal readers. One of the best diets in the world is the Paleo diet, which is currently being used by millions of people worldwide for more than 2.5 million years. Not only does it have endless health benefits, but it can also help in losing weight and reducing the symptoms of many diseases. This book is a comprehensive and concise book dedicated to embracing the Paleo diet and lifestyle.

We will guide readers through a successful diet in an easy to understand and straightforward format.

Nutrition specialist and fitness enthusiast, Emma Vickens has been in the business for over ten years and is still driven by the same objective, which is to share as much of her knowledge as she can to people so that they can live a happier, longer and healthier life.

She firmly believes that you are what you eat and adopting healthy habits is life changing. Vickens works with a holistic approach to health where she puts her focus on natural remedies through food and nutrients. She knows, through her experiences, that changing habits; the way you eat, the way you think about nutrition are a difficult challenge, but she also knows that achieving it is far more rewarding.

Her most valuable advice will always be to eat organic fruits and vegetables, free raised meat and pure drinking water. Emma believes that Mother Nature gave us everything we need to live a healthy life, and that society is, by all means, killing us. By the use of conservatives, protein meat, chemicals in fruits and vegetables, all of it is full of unhealthy products that provoke early diseases, weak body, and low-energy levels.

She recently took the road to explore different cultures and was educated by the ones who grow their food in every continent. From village to village she has experienced the habits and healthy diet of every culture that only a few people continue to follow. Mixing her knowledge with what she has learned became a real opportunity to share it.

For the past ten years, she has been working as a private nutritionist, offering cooking classes and speaking publicly. The last step in her journey is to write down on paper what she knows so she can reach as many people as she can, hoping you will be inspired and live a healthier and happier life.

INTRODUCTION

In today's world, millions of people are consuming an unhealthy diet on a daily basis and as a result, many people are suffering from physical, mental, and health problems. The Paleo diet has been used for years now and has proven to be extremely effective. Many people have begun experiencing health benefits within thirty days of implementing it.

All over the world, more people are trying out the Paleo diet thanks to its authenticity and effectiveness. This diet stands out, especially when compared to other diets that have appeared within the past few years.

In this book, we will explain how to adopt a complete Paleo lifestyle so you can feel healthy, increase levels of energy, and even lose weight. With the "Paleo diet: the 4 weeks challenge", you can begin enjoying better health and overall life – all while decreasing your chances of suffering from diseases such as cancer, cardiovascular diseases, diabetes, and other modern health problems. Not only is the information in this book going to assist you in making a successful transition to the Paleo lifestyle, but it also consists of amazing recipes that taste great and are very easy to prepare.

This book also includes detailed information on how you can start the Paleo challenge. This is a scientifically proven diet and challenge that only takes 21 days to change your daily eating habits and become a healthier you. This 4 weeks challenge has been designed to guide you as you learn to adapt to this new habit progressively and try unique recipes every day.

This is the perfect time for you ***to download your workbook*** and begin planning your challenge. The workbook is completely for free.

To do so, go on my website:

www.emmavickens.com

and download your freebie + a little bonus.

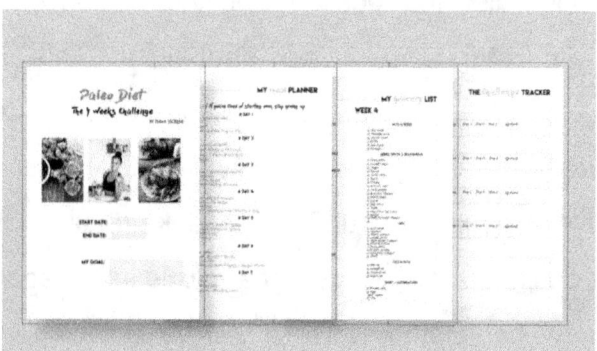

Through her books, she hopes to give you enough content that will enable you to grow on your own. Her experiences have made it possible and she is extremely happy to share her personalized recipes. The diet plans she has created for years have proven to work for thousands of individuals. Cooking can be an easy task with the right ingredients, tools, and instructions and this is the challenge she decided to overpass. Eat clean and easy for a healthier and happier life.

CHAPTER 1: WHAT IS THE PALEO DIET?

History

The concept of a Paleo diet can be traced back to a book that was published by Walter Voegtlin, a leading gastroenterologist. During 1985, the ideas in the book were further on developed by Melvin Konner and Stanley Eaton, and then popularize by Loren Cordain. During 2013, the Paleo diet was the most popular searched for weight loss technique in Google.

The Paleo diet is one of many weight loss diets that have been promoted during the past few years, but the difference is that it has many health benefits and actually works. The diet also draws on the nature and conspiracy theory about the way nutritional research and studies, which don't support the supposed advantages of the Paleo diet, are regulated and controlled by a harmful food industry.

The Paleo diet, also known as the Paleolithic and caveman diet is based on foods assumed to only be available to Paleolithic humans. There is a wide range in the way the Paleo diet is explained. It consists of vegetables, nuts, roots, fruits, and even organ meats. On the other hand, it excludes certain types of food like dairy products, legumes, salt, coffee, processed oils, and alcohol. The diet is mainly based on not consuming modern processed foods and foods that people started eating after the Neolithic Revolution. The main reason why many people opt for the Paleo diet is because it improves health and helps in reducing the symptoms of many health conditions, especially digestive disorders.

Admittedly, the word "caveman" can make it sound like a strange fad diet, but believe me, it isn't at all. During the past 300,000 years, humans consumed the best whole foods such as plants and seafood because they consist of the nutrients and minerals that our body has evolved to survive on.

Agriculture first started during the last ten thousand years, a small fraction of our history of evolution- and there hasn't been sufficient time along with evolutionary pressure for people to adapt to modern foods such as sugar and wheat. It really isn't a coincidence that modern diseases such as autoimmune disorders and obesity have accompanied the international spread and popularity of industrialized food.

To put it in a simpler way, Paleo provides an effective model for living in a healthy holistic way. The Paleo diet encourages foods that are whole and consists of high amounts of nutrients and vitamins that your body needs. It isn't an elimination diet like many people think it is. On the contrary, the Paleo diet recommends indulging in your favorite unhealthy food on an occasional basis but this is going to be explained in more detail in the book.

By eliminating many of the different causes of diseases, especially allergies and different types of autoimmune disorder, also with processed products that are a result of modern manufacturing, this is going to have many benefits on your body, both physically and mentally. By following the Paleo diet, the human body will be able to effectively detox from unhealthy foreign substances. After it detoxes, it will be able to naturally reset all the different basic functions that make the processes of eating, breathing, and even moving effortlessly in a healthy body. In other words, the Paleo diet focuses on returning back to the basics. It is a diet that works with our genetics, not the other way around.

The Paleo diet strongly takes into consideration the wisdom of our ancestors, whether it is from our Paleolithic ancestors or completely remote native ones who were untouched by any western effects or diseases. The Paleo diet focuses on what they ate and the way they lived. Most of the meals and ingredients that our ancestors consumed aren't even available in the supermarkets right now and the Paleo diet provides guidance in completely avoiding these products, especially that they have more harmful effects on the mind and body.

When you look all around you, you are going to find that the human body is assaulted on all different sides by many things in our environment, like pollutants that are extremely toxic to our regular chemical processes. This also includes all the different contaminants that are found in what we consume along with the various additives that are found in meals that our body finds it difficult to operate without when they are eliminated from our diet. Our body should be able to reach healthy and vibrant wellness completely on it owns, often without the assist of medicine or surgery. However, due to all the unhealthy food and drinks that we consume, there are many people who are suffering from health issues and they don't know that this can be mainly contributed to the food we eat.

The Paleo diet advises to completely avoid certain things such as grains, gluten, dairy that is low in fat and pasteurize, corn, soy, and even meals with high quantities of sugar. Instead, it recommends filling up on meat that is grass fed from ruminants such as cattle, lamb, and goats. Try as much as possible to consume pastured chicken, seafood, and wild caught fish as much as possible.

Other than encouraging healthy components in your diet, Paleo also attempts to solve serious diseases that are caused by living in the modern world. Unlike other types of diet, it doesn't just encourage to cut or add on what you eat. The Paleo diet also strongly focuses on aspects such as stress reduction, engaging with your community, exercising and staying fit, exposure to the environment and honoring the circadian rhythms of the body. Therefore, there is a lot more to the Paleo diet than simply changing what you eat or drink.

The Paleo diet has proven to be really effective for people who want to lose weight. A study conducted by the Edith Cowan University (ECU) proved that. Researchers assigned thirty-nine healthy women on a Paleo or Australian diet for 4 weeks to assess how much weight they are going to lose. Meals consumed on the Paleo diet were eggs, fruits, vegetables, and lean meats whereas dairy and grains were completely prohibited. Angelo Genoni, one of the lead researchers in the study, found that women who were following the Paleo diet were losing an average of 2 kilograms more throughout the phase than the other diet group. Genoni also explained that both groups ended up losing weight throughout the testing phase, but the Paleo group ended up losing 4.3% of their overall body weight in contrast to 1.6% that was lost by the advisable dietary strategy group. Those who were following the standard diet were asked to increase their vegetables, fruit, and whole grain consumption, decrease fat consumption and eat dairy products that are low in fat. The research is currently published in the MDPI journal.

The Paleo diet, with its focus on the consumption of meat, is amenable to a high intake of protein. This is why other high protein diets, like the Atkins diet, are really popular for losing weight and a lot of research has been conducted on them.

Some of the reasons why the protein intake in the Paleo diet is beneficial are:

1/ When the body consumes protein, the brain transmits a hormone that informs the stomach to stop drinking or eating. Research shows that individuals who consume a significant amount of protein (thirty to fifty percent) in their diet aren't going to want food, especially snacks, for longer amounts of time. What exactly leads to this isn't understood until now.

2/ Eating protein leads to diet-induced thermogenesis (DIT), a change in the body's metabolism, which assists in increasing the quantity of weight loss for individuals who want to diet. However, one of the main types of protein that leads to this change is milk proteins, something that isn't included in the Paleo diet.

3/ The meat's texture and associated effort by the jaws result in a higher satiation sense.

4/ Protein and fat take longer to break down and digest, causing dieters to feel full for long periods of time.

5/ Simple carbohydrates and sugars that are specifically processed cause peaks in insulin and even crashes. This results in the body of dieters reacting with a mental craving to eat, and a physical feeling of being tired or shaky. The ups and downs that take place in the body impact the way the body processes and saves the fats that are found in the bloodstream.

However, there is something that I really want you to understand: we aren't precisely copying caveman diets. Many Paleo dieters prefer to opt for super low carbohydrates, whereas others like me are happy to indulge in a baked potato every now and then. The Paleo diet is big enough to include various approaches, but the main codes of ancestral eating are the same and they are:

Eat whole, nourishing, nutrients packed and unprocessed meals. Prioritize meats that are grass fed and meats that are pastured, seafood that is wild-caught, and vegetables. Fruits and seeds should be consumed in moderation. Try as much as possible to avoid meals that will harm you by causing inflammation, harming your guts, or derailing the overall metabolic process. Completely abstain from any meals that consist of gluten-packed grains, sugar, and legumes.

The next chapters are going to get into more detail about what you should eat and avoid.

CHAPTER 2 : BENEFITS OF THE PALEO DIET

This chapter is going to explain in detail all the different benefits of the Paleo diet.

BENEFIT #1 | HEALTHIER CELLS

You probably don't know this, but every cell in your body consists of saturated and unsaturated fat. Also, cells depend on a balance between the two of them to properly transmit messages. The Paleo diet provides a regular and the perfect balance of fats as it suggests the two types of fats in healthy ones whereas other diets either limit both or one of them.

Scientific proof

Also called polyunsaturated fatty acids, omega-3 fatty acids have an important role in the way the brain functions, along with its development and growth – *Harvard University and Maryland University.*

BENEFIT #2 | HEALTHIER BRAIN AND CARDIOVASCULAR HEALTH

One of the best protein and fat sources comes from cold water fish, especially salmon. Salmon fat includes significant amounts of omega 3 fatty acid which the average diet doesn't include. This is an issue because omega 3 fatty acids consist of DHA, which is greatly beneficial for the eyes, brain development, and heart. Other sources of omega 3 can be found in pasture-raised meats and eggs.

Scientific proof
Studies indict that inflammation is the main reason behind cardiovascular disease. The best thing about the Paleo diet is that most of the meals are anti-inflammatory so your risk will decrease. The DHA found in omega 3 fatty acids promotes healthy cardiovascular health.

BENEFIT #3 | LESS FAT AND MORE MUSCLE

The Paleo diet heavily depends on animal flesh and this includes healthy protein. This is anabolic protein and is mainly used for building new cells and muscle mass. When you have more muscle, your metabolism is going to work better. This is because muscles need the energy to function effectively. This enables your body to send energy to the muscle cells instead of all the energy being sent to fat cells. By decreasing fat cells and increasing muscle cells, an extra energy is going to go to glycogen found in your muscles instead of triglycerides that are found in fat cells.

Scientific proof
Genetics results in people having higher rates of metabolism than other people. However, muscle mass is an essential factor to take into consideration in finding out your BMR. Your muscles are more active and need more energy, so if you have a higher amount of muscles instead of fats, this means that you have a higher BMR. – *mckinley.illinois.edu*

BENEFIT #4 | BETTER GUT HEALTH

Sugar, processed fats, and other junk lead to issues and inflammation in the digestive system. Unfortunately, eating junk and being under a lot of stress leads to even more problems. For example, leaky gut syndrome is a digestive disorder that involves the breach of the intestinal walls and whatever you consume leaks out of the intestines. Obviously, you don't want this to happen to you and you can prevent this and other digestive disorders by following the Paleo diet.

Scientific proof
The amount of blood sugar that is found in a highly refined carbohydrates meal, such as white rice and French fries increases amounts of inflammatory messages in the body such as cytokines.

BENEFIT #5 | LIFE'S CIRCLE

The Paleo diet encourages consuming eggs and meats that are pasture raised. This means that animals should be able to roam in the grass throughout their entire lives. Ideally, chickens and other animals like cows are going to wander the pasture together because this leads to synergy.

In nature, chickens follow cows and consume the larvae found in cow pies. Naturally, cow pies are broken up which also fertilizes grass which is food the cow can consume. This natural diet is excellent for animals but it also provides you with a long list of nutrients when you consume them because of their healthy diet. This is definitely the circle of life at its best.

Scientific proof
Eggs from hens that are pastured can consist as much as ten times more amounts of omega 3 than eggs from hens in factories. – *eatwild.com*

BENEFIT #6 | GETTING THE NEEDED VITAMINS AND MINERALS

The Paleo diet encourages eating what is called the "rainbow". Vegetables are an important component of the diet and it is advisable to consume different vegetables based on the season. The various colors of vegetables depend on the nutrients they consist of. By consuming the rainbow, you get all the vitamins and nutrients you need!

Scientific proof
Vegetables are essential nutrients' sources, such as potassium, foliate, vitamin A and C. - *choosemyplate.gov*

BENEFIT #7 | BETTER DIGESTION

The Paleo diet encourages consuming food that your body has adapted the capability to digest over thousands of years. There aren't questions whether you can tolerate starch or not. Your ancestors were perfectly able to thrive off and digest these foods. If you're having digestion issue, try a Paleo diet for thirty days and trust me, you are going to feel better.

Scientific proof
Fermented foods, whether it is sauerkraut or yogurt, are increasingly being considered to be a benefit to the gut- and benefit not only your digestive health but promote weight loss- *nutritionletter.tufts.edu*

BENEFIT #8 | LESS ALLERGIES

The Paleo diet encourages you to avoid foods that are allergens to certain societies. Many people are not able to digest seeds and dairy and this is the main reason why the diet recommends that you eliminate these foods for a month, except if the milk is completely raw.

Many people are against the diet because we don't consume whole grains. But this isn't true at all. The truth is that grains don't really do the job, so we prevent eating high amounts of whole grains most of the time. If you play sports, then it's a good idea to consume oats every now and then.

Scientific Proof
Reported consumption of raw milk was inversely connected to asthma"-*jacionline.org*

BENEFIT #9 | HIGHER ENERGY LEVELS

Ever wonder the reason why energy drinks have become really popular during the last few years? It's because everyone is consuming a crappy diet.

A typical breakfast looks something like this: a coffee high in sugar with a muffin or cream cheese croissant. Not only is this going to lead to many health issues like diabetes, but it won't keep you full and provide the energy levels you need to get through your day. With the Paleo diet, you will be able to strategically select the right foods for any type of occasion and make sure you have sufficient energy levels.

Scientific proof

Eating foods that consist of a low index of glycemic-where sugars are absorbed really slowly- can assist you in preventing the lag in levels of energy that usually takes place after consuming refined starches and sugars that are quickly absorbed.

BENEFIT #10 | WEIGHT LOSS

The Paleo diet consists of meals which have low amounts of carbohydrates by design. Simply eliminating processed foods will drastically decrease your carb intake in order to promote weight loss. By limiting carbohydrate to around exercise times, you will prevent unwanted fat gain which is usually a result of excess carbohydrates.

Scientific proof

Many food types that increase the risk of diabetes-refined drinks and drinks full of sugar among them- are important factors in gaining weight. - *Harvard University.*

CHAPTER 3: A LITTLE MORE ABOUT PALEO DIET

The Paleo diet involves spending more time preparing food and choosing it. Not only this but for individuals who are worried about where the meat, fish, fruits, vegetables, and other types of food came from, there can be a lot of work involved in finding and creating relationships with local farmers and butchers. Once this is done, you are going to have to accept that you will be paying visits to these places on a regular basis. This is because unlike other types of diet, you need to make sure that everything is fresh and isn't frozen for long periods of time.

Let's have a look at what is and isn't allowed to eat when doing the paleo diet:

WHAT TO EAT:

Fresh fruits

Grass-fed meats

Fresh vegetables

Seafood & Fish

Nuts

Eggs

Seeds

Healthy oils (olive, walnut, flaxseed, macadamia, avocado, coconut)

WHAT NOT TO EAT

Refined sugar

Legumes (peanuts also)

Dairy

Processed, Candy or junk food

Potatoes

Processed foods

Cereal grains

Too salty foods

Refined vegetable oils

Here is the main list of what you should avoid when following the paleo diet:

Dairy - anything but goat milk products

Soft drinks - anything with gas and with high amounts or even low amounts of added sugar, sirop. (Coke, peps, etc.)

Fruit Juices - unfortunately they are also high in sugar (fructose) and will be bad for your diet.

Grains - You must avoid everything that contains grains.

Legumes - here is the list of the ones to avoid

All beans

Peas

Snow peas

Chickpeas

Sugar snap peas

Peanut butter

Peanuts

Miso

Lupins

Lentils

Mesquite

All soybean products and derivatives

Tofu

Any other beans.

Artificial Sweeteners - All sweeteners are against paleo diet, here is the full list of the main categories in alphabotical ordor:

Acesulfame potassium

Aspartame

Aspartame-acesulfame salt

Cyclamate

Calcium cyclamate

Erythritol

Glycerol

Glycyrrhizin

Hydrogenated starch hydrolysate (HSH)

Isomalt

Lactitol

Maltitol

Mannitol

Neotame

Polydextrose

Saccharin

Sorbitol

Steviol glycoside

Sucralose

Tagatose

Xylitol

If you read "artificial on the label you can avoid it.

Fatty Meats - there are meats that have to be avoided in paleo diet, not all but the ones below:

Hot dogs

Not free raised meat (any kind)

Any kind of meat from fast foods

Salty Foods - they tend to add so much salt in the list below, therefore you have to stay away from them too:

Ketchup

French fries

Salted peanuts

Pringles

Chips

Bretzels

Cookies

Brownies

Pastries

Starchy Vegetables - (Potatoes, Beets, Yucca, Yam, Sweet potatoes, Batata)

Energy Drinks - as a general comment, energyy drinks are bad for the health and certainly not approved by the paleo diet. (red bull, ,monster, and so on)

Alcohol - cavemen did not know the process of making alcohol therefore the paleo diet doesn't approve it either. I am sorry, you will have to avoid it as well.

To come back to what I previously mentioned above about having to look for better products yourself. I personally enjoy all the different relationships I made with suppliers and butchers. Believe it or not, I have also established greater bonds with individuals over meal preparation and cooking.

Sure, you obviously can't whip up a meal in minimal times, but why not make food an integral part of your life. This is something that you may encounter on a regular basis throughout your daily life, so no matter how someone likes the subject of food, you know that you can share this with them on some level. One of the main things I am trying to do with this book is to give you different ways to turn something that might look inconvenient to you in the beginning into something that isn't really that stressful or big.

CHAPTER 4 : INTRODUCTION TO THE CHALLENGE

If you have decided to follow the Paleo diet, then this is excellent news as you are on the journey to a healthier and better life. The main purpose of this chapter is to fully prepare you for the Paleo challenge so that you can enjoy your journey and overcome any difficulties you may face along the way.

Preparing yourself

Clean your kitchen

Collect all the "no" foods such as grains, vegetable oils, cheese, packaged foods, unhealthy preservatives, you understand- and throw them in the trash. This will benefit you more because it is easier to avoid any temptation when it is actually isn't there.

However, if you choose to follow baby steps, then this is completely fine as well. Perhaps you can eliminate dairy during the first week, get rid of refined grains the second week, and then grains the week after, and so on. Either way, make sure that your kitchen consists of whole foods before you start your Paleo challenge so you have a lot to diet.

Follow your motivation

One of the main reasons many people follow the Paleo diet is to assist with medical problems, like autoimmune and gut problems, intolerances, and allergies. Some people just want to feel healthier on a daily basis and believe that this is the healthiest way to diet. Your reason is going to determine the rules you follow and what exactly you would like to be careful about. It is essential that you follow your personal guidelines for the first thirty days, and be really strict about it. You need thirty days to begin noticing health benefits.

Implement the 85/15 rule

During the first month, many professionals advocate the 85/15 concept, meaning that 85% of the time you are following the Paleo diet, and the 15% is for non-Paleo meals. This can be anything from a granola bar, cocktails with your friends, to a hamburger. Make sure that you pay close attention to the way you feel after you reintroduce new things to your diet. For example, if you consume ice cream and then wake up the next day feeling bloated, your future discomfort is definitely not worth it.

Cook

Due to the fact that Paleo is based on whole and fresh foods, it is a lot easier to prepare meals in your own kitchen instead of a restaurant where it is difficult to control which ingredients should be used. Take advantage of this opportunity to try out new foods. Give yourself a challenge. Why not purchase the weirdest looking fruit and vegetable and look up how to prepare it. If you're worried to prepare any of the recipes in this book or think they're difficult? Why not challenge yourself and prepare them anyway?

Expect setbacks

It is completely normal to start following a Paleo diet and then go back into your normal habits. However, you should never take this as a failure and only as a learning process. The most important thing is for you not to repeat this mistake again. I recommend finding people like you who are following the diet through social media sites or forums, and then connect with them to stay on track and for support.

Decode labels

You know how to avoid doughnuts and crackers, but some ingredients are not Paleo and you might be surprised to know that. For example, soy sauce, different types of marinades, and dried fruit without any added sugars. It is essential to read the list of ingredients properly when you are buying anything.

Change your oil

Instead of opting for canola or corn, use coconut oil instead. Lard is an excellent option as well. These saturated fats are really healthy to cook, are more stable, and aren't going to oxidize when they are heated. For a cold application, walnut, olive, and avocado are all great choices.

Eat meat

Many people don't include meat in their diet because they think that it is harmful to their health. The truth is that you can eat meat, but the key here is to make sure that it's good and high quality. When you begin your Paleo diet, this is going to be the time to say goodbye to unhealthy processed meats like bologna and salami. Wild meats such as bison and boar are a perfect choice, along with meats that are pasture fed and poultry. Your last choice should be lean meat that is grain-fed. When it comes to seafood, choose wild-caught fish as much as you can. I personally recommend sustainable and low-mercury options.

Satisfy your cravings

Completely giving up sugar is really difficult in the beginning. If you like having dessert after dinner, then you substitute the cookies or chocolate cake with fresh fruit. With time, you are going to start getting used to this and so will your taste buds.

Don't worry so much about eating out

Brunches or lunches with your friends are still doable when you go on the Paleo diet. It only requires some ingredient sleuthing. The first thing you should do is look at the restaurant's menu before you go there and choose one or two choices that you can easily "paleo-ize". This could be wild salmon and broccoli. If you're ordering rice pilaf, for example, ask them to double the serving of vegetables. You should never feel shy to ask any questions about how things can be prepared and ask for changes if needed.

Here are some tips that are going to help you succeed when you begin the Paleo diet:-

✓ **Follow the Paleo diet as closely as you can**. Yes, there will be the occasional detour here and there, and having something you are allowed to can be worth the treat. However, it is essential to keep things moving in the correct direction, especially if you are suffering from a health issue. This means completely avoiding things such as gluten, processed sugar, and inflammatory food as much as possible.

✓ **Simple does the trick.** Cooking can sometimes become an overwhelming activity when we become wrapped up in time consuming and difficult recipes. This is why you will notice that all the recipes included in the book are simple.

✓ **Make sure it's crazy delicious.** Many people think that the Paleo diet is about depriving your body, and that everything we eat is basically meat with some broccoli on the side. There are many times where people told me, ''the reason I can't get on a Paleo diet is because there will be nothing to eat''. This isn't true at all and you will find that the recipes mentioned in this book are extremely tasty and unbelievably good for you.

Reasons why people fail

You could have just started your Paleo journey and find it a challenge to shift from your old lifestyle to a new one. You might also be a veteran to the Paleo diet, but occasionally find yourself pick away here and there on chocolate or bread. Even worse, you could feel that you are eating right and doing everything you can, but you still aren't experiencing any results when it comes to weight loss, more energy, or enhanced general health. These are all things that I hear on a regular basis and the good news is that you can completely avoid and overcome this.

Like any other new adjustment and change to your life, there are going to be obstacles and issues here and there knocking at your door. Unfortunately, change isn't something that is easy to accomplish and needs determination and hard work. The change in your life is going to test your ability to remain committed and motivated. Even though it isn't going to be easy in the beginning, I can promise you that you will reap the benefits.

So why do many people fail to regularly follow the diet or never see excellent results? This can be really different for everyone, but here are some common reasons and how you can overcome them.

Technical reasons

These technical reasons are usually the main reason why many people fail to accomplish positive health results even though they strictly follow the diet and do everything the right way. There are many conflicting and confusing information about the Paleo diet and many individuals are led to make positive changes based on wrong information that isn't beneficial for them on the long run.

Not enough salt

There's no denial that large quantities of salt can be an issue, but eliminating salt entirely is harmful as well. I've come across many people who began having problems with low blood pressure when they started the Paleo diet. This can be easily solved by adding some natural sea salt on occasion to your food. The issue is that many people think that the Paleo diet is about following our ancestors in every single thing that they do. One thing they don't know is that our ancestors probably went a long way to get the little additional sodium in the food.

Not enough carbohydrates

Many people who follow the Paleo diet become carb-phobic and connect carbohydrates with quick fat gain. We need to keep in mind that gaining weight and fat is a lot more complicated and that we are perfectly adapted to function on carbohydrates. This is why many individuals limit their intake of carbohydrates to extremely low amounts. Even when sufficient fat amounts are consumed for the low amount of carbohydrates, putting a limit on the number of carbohydrates consumed can result in strong cravings and even binding on sugar and unhealthy foods.

Many people fear starchy carbohydrates as they are concentrated. If we begin with the concept that carbohydrates aren't really that bad, we can begin seeing why it isn't realistic to be worried about concentrated sources such as starchy vegetables. The conclusion is that carbohydrates shouldn't be feared at all, but carbohydrates from toxic sources such as grains and processed sugars should.

Not enough fat

Again in attempting to copy our Paleolithic ancestors, many people are still convinced that fat has to be consumed in limited amounts. These people think that wild animals are extremely lean and our ancestors never consumed fat. However, what many people overlook is that lean animals have a lot of fat tissues surrounding their organs and between their muscles. Modern research demonstrates that saturated fat is an excellent source of non-toxic and healthy energy whereas lean protein is an issue.

As you can see, many people limit their fat and carbohydrate intake, which is our two main fuel sources, and increase their intake of more lean protein or eat fewer calories. For those who consume low amounts of calories, they will usually feel hungry and their levels of energy usually fall. Indulge in healthy

49

saturated fat from natural sources and non-toxic carbohydrates.

Not enough nutritious meals

This issue is not really that popular, but it still takes place. In the modern world, consuming a non-toxic diet isn't enough and vitamins and minerals are required to deal with the stress and negative environmental factors surrounding us. This means that vegetables and poultry on a daily basis aren't enough. You have to strive to consume meals like fresh fish that is wild caught, seafood, bone marrow, and different fresh vegetables.

Too many fruits

Fruits are definitely natural, but many of them consist of high amounts of fructose, which can become toxic when eaten in large quantities. Due to fruits being loaded with potassium, fiber, and other sources of natural anti-oxidants we think we can consume as much as we want, although it doesn't necessarily mean that the fructose in them isn't that toxic.

A couple of fruit pieces every day isn't an issue whatsoever, but eating large quantities could be the main reason why many people fail to lose weight even if they go on the Paleo diet. Many vegetables, once digested are transformed into glucose, therefore our body already gets the amount of glucose needed. The fruits should remain essential for other nutritional benefits such as vitamins.

Forgetting about other lifestyle aspects

Lifestyle factors have a really important role and shouldn't be neglected. The three main factors are exercise, stress relief, and getting adequate sleep.

Failure to maintain healthy habits can greatly hinder your success. Not sleeping properly or having poor sleep quality can be harmful and there isn't an amount of healthy food that is going to make up for this.

Not properly committing

Implementing the diet only to a certain extent is something that many people are doing. I hear from many of my clients on a daily basis that they aren't really noticing a difference when they're seeing a switch, but we soon find out together that they aren't really committed.

I still remember when one of my friends decided to try out the diet. She was really excited about the challenge and was definitely committed from the start. A couple of weeks into it, and she began getting tempted to try out other types of food. She used to say things like what is one piece of chocolate going to really do? This might be difficult to believe, but she began feeling the consequences of this the whole week after. This includes fatigue, tummy aches, nausea, headaches, and a general feeling of being unwell.

Expensive lifestyle

I personally think it's crazy that anyone would ever consider thinking about putting a cost on their health. In fact, when when some of my clients first started following the Paleo diet, they didn't really have a big budget and were worried that they wouldn't be able to afford the high quality of food. This was also due to all the crazy stories they had heard about Paleo diet being really expensive. The truth is that the Paleo diet can consist of some meals that are more expensive than others but what I can tell you now is that the difference in prices is so minimal in comparison to what this means for your health and future that it is totally worth doing. If you review your expenses, you are going to find that you are probably spending money on things that aren't really important or crucial to your life or health anyways.

There are different ways around the higher price connected with being Paleo, but you are going to have to work a bit hard to save money here and there. One excellent way is to plant your herbs, spices, and vegetable garden. If you aren't able to do so or don't have the space for this, you should consider enrolling in a farmer's co-op. It is essential that you follow a strict meal plan. This assists me a lot, because when all your food and meals are planned, you are going to just buy what you really need and don't need to worry about spend on things that you don't need or are going to go to waste.

Finally, get connected with a farmer or butcher in your area. I go to a couple and I have to say I'm lucky to have access to great choices at reasonable prices. However, make sure to always ask them about the meat and where it comes before you buy it from them.

A couple of points to keep in mind

The Paleo lifestyle isn't a cure all and you aren't going to lose weight within a couple of days. Years of being unhealthy may have ruined your metabolism and you are probably carrying around unhealthy body fat. Switching to the Paleo diet is going to help your system, body composition, and overall health. However, the point of the Paleo diet isn't to lose as many points as you can so you can fit into that new dress or jeans you bought a couple of months ago. This nutritional diet is about enhancing your wellness and overall health- not transforming you into a size zero unhealthy model.

It is important that you stick to the diet for thirty days. For many individuals, switching to the Paleo diet isn't difficult at all. But for others, due to the unexpected decrease in dietary carbohydrates, people who are used to consuming pasta and processed sugar report that they aren't feeling well for a couple of days after going on the diet. This is also known as the "Paleo diet". If you are able to make it through this sluggishness period in the beginning, which can last for about three weeks, you are going to come to the other end feeling better than you have ever been in your life.

Eat food like a champion and never be scared to try the new recipes in this book or experience new types of food. The diet can seem a bit restrictive in the beginning, but you will soon find that the Paleo diet provides an infinite variety, nourishment, and health benefits.

RECIPES
WEEK 1

BREAKFAST OPTIONS

★   Paleo Bacon and Eggs

★   Paleo Chocolate Muffin

★   Banane et Smoothie aux baies rouges

★   Cashew Milk Hot Chocolate

★   Latte Coco with Green Tea Matcha

★   Paleo Tortilla

★   Red Fruits Crumble

LUNCH OPTIONS

★   Kale Salad

★   Paleo Quiche with Spaghetti Squash

★   Green Bean Salad

★   Scallop tartare with Mango

★   Grounded Sweet Potatoes and Spinach

★   Scallops with Zucchini & Carrots

★   Steak Tartare

SNACK OPTIONS

★ Paleo Biscuit

★ Coconut Sugar & Vanilla Baked Apple

★ Ice Coffee Coco Vanilla

★ Baked Kale Chips

★ Super Energetic Drink

★ Strawberry Sorbet

★ Sweet potatoes chips

DINNER OPTIONS

★ Basil Beef and Green Peppers Wok

★ Chicken fajitas

★ Beef & Sweet Potatoes Moussaka

★ Chicken with Spinach on Sweet Potatoes &
Eggs

★ Grilled Pork Chop

★ Chicken Curry Stir Fried Pumpkin & Smoked
Almond

★ Shrimps Skewer with Citrus Salad

DAY 1

BREAKFAST: PALEO BACON AND EGGS

Makes 1 Serving

Ingredients

- 3 Eggs - whole
- 2 Bacon slices
- 1 tbsp. Olive oil
- 1 tbsp. Pesto
- 1 tbsp. Tapenade

Directions

1. Gently place 2 eggs in a pot of boiling water.

2. Remove the first egg after 3 minutes – soft-boiled egg

3. Remove the second egg after 10 minutes – hard-boiled egg.

4. Cook the bacon in a skillet until crispy.

5. Break an egg into a bowl and mix it with tapenade and pesto.

6. Cook the mixture to the skillet

7. Serve immediately and enjoy!

LUNCH: KALE SALAD
Makes 2 Servings

Ingredients

- 8 leaves of kale – chopped
- 1 tbsp. lemon juice – freshly squeezed
- 3 tbsp. vegetable oil
- 1 carrot – julienned cut
- 1 apple – sliced
- 1 tbsp. oilseeds (hazelnuts, almonds or cashews)
- 1 tbsp. of seeds (sesame, flax)
- Nuts of choice (almonds, walnuts, cashews, etc.)

Directions

1. Rinse the leaves and remove the central ribs of the kale
2. Chop the kale cabbage coarsely
3. Prepare the salad dressing with mashed oilseed
4. Stir in the dressing with the chopped kale cabbage for roughly 1-2 minutes until well-combined.
5. Add the carrots and apples and mix
6. Sprinkle with flax seeds and sesame
7. Top with nuts of choice – optional
8. Serve and enjoy!

SNACK: COCONUT SUGAR & VANILLA BAKED APPLE
Makes 2 Serving

Ingredients

- 2 apples – organic
- 1 tbsp. Coconut sugar
- 1 tbsp. Coconut oil – organic
- 1 pinch of vanilla powder

Directions
1. Preheat oven to 375 F Degrees
2. Rinse the apples and remove the cores.
3. Mix the coconut sugar, coconut oil, and vanilla powder
4. Add the mixture to fill in the apples
5. Bake for 30 minutes until golden
6. Serve warm and enjoy!

DINNER: BASIL BEEF AND GREEN PEPPERS WOK

Makes 4 Servings

Ingredients

- 400g of Beef – sliced thinly
- 3 Green Peppers
- 1 tbsp. Olive oil – extra virgin
- 1 onion – chopped
- 1 bunch Basil –chopped thinly
- 1 garlic clove – sliced
- 1 tbsp. Arrowroot Powder (dissolved in 4 tbsp. water)

Directions

1. Slice the beef into thin slices and set apart
2. Wash the green peppers and cut into strips – remove the stalk and seeds
3. In a medium-sized wok, drizzle olive oil and place over medium heat
4. Prepare the onion and fry in wok until softened
5. Stir in the beef and peppers and cook until the meat is brown
6. Add the garlic clove

7. While the meat is cooking, slice the basil leaves thinly and add to the wok

8. Once the peppers soften, add the arrowroot powder mixture

9. Stir until you achieve a smooth texture

10. Remove wok from heat

11. Serve immediately and enjoy!

DAY 2

BREAKFAST: PALEO CHOCOLATE MUFFIN
Makes 4 Servings

Ingredients

- 2 Medium Bananas – Ripened
- 2 Eggs - whole
- ½ cup Coconut Flour
- 1 tbsp. Raw Honey - organic
- 1 tbsp. Bicarbonate Soda
- 1 tbsp. Cacao Nibs
- 1 tsp. Apple Cider Vinegar

Directions

1. Remove peels and cut the bananas into pieces
2. Place in a medium bowl
3. Add the remaining ingredients into the bowl and mix until well-blended
4. Pour the banana mixture into muffin pans
5. Sprinkle the cocoa nibs on top
6. Bake at 400 F degrees for 15 minutes

LUNCH: PALEO QUICHE WITH SPAGHETTI SQUASH
Makes 4 Servings

Ingredients

- 1 Sweet Potato
- 3 cups of Spaghetti Squash
- 4 Eggs - whole
- 200 ml coconut milk
- Salt, Pepper, Nutmeg – to taste

Directions

1. Peel the sweet potato and cut into thin slices (about 2mm) using a mandolin slicer
2. Preheat oven to 350 Degrees F
3. Place baking paper into a mold and add the sweet potato slices to cover the entire mold
4. In a medium bowl mix the eggs, coconut milk, and spaghetti squash until combined
5. Season with salt, pepper, and a pinch of nutmeg
6. Pour the mixture over the sweet potatoes and place in the oven to bake for 35 minutes
7. Serve warm and enjoy!

SNACK: PALEO BISCUIT
For 10 biscuit

Ingredients

- ¼ cup Hazelnut Puree
- ¼ cup Almond Flour
- ¼ cup Almond Powder
- ½ cup Raw Honey – organic
- 1 dash Salt
- 1 tsp Ground Cinnamon
- 1 dash of Sesame Seeds

Directions

1. Preheat oven to 350° F
2. Combine the hazelnut puree, hazelnut flour, and almond powder and mix
3. Add honey, cinnamon powder and salt, mix until combined
4. Craft the dough into a cookie form and place separately on a baking sheet
5. Sprinkle the sesame seeds to the biscuit dough
6. Bake for 10-15 minutes until golden
7. Let it cool and enjoy!

DINNER: CHICKEN FAJITAS
Makes 4-6 Servings

Ingredients

- 1 pound chicken breast - cut into strips
- 1 Bell pepper - stripped
- 2 Onions - chopped
- 3 Garlic cloves - minced
- 3 tbsp. Lemon juice – freshly squeezed
- 1 tbsp. Coconut oil
- Oregano
- Cumin
- Coriander

Directions

1. In a large bowl, add the chicken strips, bell peppers, onions, garlic, lemon juice and spices and mix until combined.

2. Let the mixture marinate in the refrigerator for at least 4 hours – the longer, the tastier

3. Place coconut oil into your frying pan and set over medium heat

4. Add the mixture and cook for 20 minutes – stirring frequently

5. One the chicken in fully cooked, remove from heat

6. Serve warm and enjoy!

DAY 3

BREAKFAST: BANANA & RED BERRIES SMOOTHIE
Makes 1 Serving

Ingredients

- 1 handful of Red Berries
- 1 banana – ripened
- 1 tbsp. Raw Honey – organic
- 1 cup of Ice

Directions

1. Place all ingredients into a blender or Vitamix
2. Blend until you achieve liquid results
3. Serve immediately and enjoy!

Bonus idea: Add tbsp. of coconut milk, to taste.

LUNCH: GREEN BEAN SALAD
Makes 2 Servings

Ingredients

- 1 cup Green Beans
- 10 Dried Tomatoes
- 2 Eggs - whole
- 5 pickles or Cucumber
- 1 tsp. Apple Cider Vinegar
- 3 tbsp. of coconut oil
- 1 shallot
- Salt
- Pepper

Directions

1. Wash the beans and remove stalks
2. Steam for 15 minutes, let cool
3. Boil the eggs for 10 minutes – for hard-boiled eggs results
4. Cut the dried tomatoes, pickles or cucumber, and shallot into slices
5. Remove the egg shelves, chop into pieces and place on top.

SNACK: ICE COFFEE COCO VANILLA
Makes 2 Servings

Ingredients

- 2 tbsp Coffee
- 1 tbsp. Coconut sugar
- 1 tbsp. Vanilla extract
- 1 tbsp. Coconut cream
- 1 cup of Ice Cubes

Directions

1. Make the coffee, add sugar and mix.

2. Let it cool and place in the refrigerator for 30 minutes to 1 hour

3. Pour the coffee into the blondor

4. Add vanilla extract, coconut cream, and ice cubes

5. Mix until well-combined

6. Serve immediately and enjoy!

DINNER: BEEF & SWEET POTATOES MOUSSAKA

Makes 2 Servings

Ingredients

- 8 oz. of Ground Beef
- 2 sweet potatoes
- 1 onion –sliced
- 1 eggplant
- 1 cup tomato sauce
- 2 tbsp. parsley
- 2 tbsp. coconut oil
- 1 tsp. dried mint
- 1 tsp. nutmeg
- 1 tsp. cinnamon
- 1 tsp. ground garlic

Directions

1. Preheat oven to 425 ° F
2. Poke holes in the eggplant with a fork
3. Place the eggplant in aluminum foil and bake for 40 minutes, or until tender
4. Cut lengthwise and remove flesh
5. Cut the sweet potatoes into slice and sprinkle with cinnamon

6. Bake at 425 Degrees F for 15 minutes

7. In a skillet, cook the ground beef

8. Add the garlic, onions, dried mint, nutmeg and eggplant with the beef and continue to cook

9. Pour the tomato sauce and chopped parsley and reduce to low heat

10. Add coconut oil to a lasagna dish

11. Place 1/3 of the meat mixture and one layer of sweet potatoes

12. Continue to repeat the process to create a second layer

13. Cover the top layer with sweet potatoes

14. Place the dish in the oven at 425 ° for 10 minutes

15. Remove from the oven

16. Serve warm and enjoy!

Day 4

BREAKFAST: CASHEW MILK HOT CHOCOLATE
Makes 2 Servings

Ingredients

- 2 cups of cashew milk
- 1 tbsp. Raw Cacao Powder
- 3 tbsp. of Agave Syrup
- ½ tsp. Ground Cinnamon

Directions

1. Heat milk cashew in a saucepan.
2. Stir in the raw cocoa powder, agave syrup, and cinnamon powder
3. Whisk until well-combined
4. Serve immediately and enjoy!

LUNCH: SCALLOP TARTARE WITH MANGO

Makes 2 Servings

Ingredients

- 5 scallops
- 1 mango
- 1 Lime
- 2 tbsp. olive oil
- 1 pinch of pink pepper
- 1 half onion
- Chive
- Salt
- Pepper

Directions

1. Clean the scallops and discard the white muscles
2. Remove the coral, wash and dry
3. Place in the refrigerator
4. Cut the mango into small cubes
5. To make the marinade: grate the lime peel, and squeeze the juice to mix with the zest
6. Add olive oil, crushed peppercorns, salt and pepper – to taste
7. Add to the mango mixture and chill for 5 minutes
8. Chop the scallops and onion into small cubes
9. Mix the marine with the chopped chives onion.
10. Serve immediately and enjoy!

SNACKS: BAKED KALE CHIPS
Makes 1-2 Servings

Ingredients

- 1 Head of Kale - washed thoroughly and dried
- 2 tbsp. Olive oil
- Sea salt, for flavor

Directions

1. Preheat oven to 175°C

2. Remove the ribs of the kale and cut into 2-inch pieces

3. Place kale on a baking sheet, drizzle with olive oil, and sprinkle with sea salt

4. Bake the kale chips for 10-15 minutes until crisp, be sure to turn the leaves every few minutes

5. Remove from oven, let it cool

6. Serve warm or cool and enjoy!

DINNER: CHICKEN WITH SPINACH ON SWEET POTATOES & EGGS

Makes 4 Servings

Ingredients

- 2 Chicken Breasts (cooked)
- 2 Sweet Potatoes
- 3 cups of Spinach
- 2 eggs – organic, whole
- 1 Onion – chopped
- 2 tbsp. Olive Oil
- 2 tsp. coconut oil
- 2 tsp. Paprika
- 1 tsp. Dried Chives
- Salt, pepper

Directions

For the Sweet Potatoes:

1. Preheat oven to 400 degrees F.
2. Rinse and cut the potatoes into eight – lengthwise
3. Place potatoes in a bowl and sprinkle with salt, pepper, and paprika
4. Pour 2 tbsp. olive oil over potatoes
5. Mix and place the potatoes on a parchment paper-covered baking sheet
6. Place in the oven for 40-45 minutes until golden brown

For the Chicken and Spinach with Onions:

1. Cut the chicken into shredded pieces
2. Pour 2 tbsp. coconut oil into a pan over medium heat.
3. Add the chicken, spinach, onions, chives and paprika
4. Sauté for 5 minutes

For the Egg:

1. In a frying pan add 1 tbsp. coconut oil in low heat
2. Cook two eggs – sunny side up

To Complete the Dish:

1. Spread sweet potatoes on a plate, then pour the chicken on top
2. Add the eggs, salt and pepper to taste.
3. Serve immediately and enjoy!

Day 5

BREAKFAST: LATTE COCO WITH GREEN TEA MATCHA
Makes 1 Serving

Ingredients

- ½ tsp. Green tea Matcha
- 1 cup Coconut milk - organic
- 1 pinch Cinnamon
- 1 teaspoon Raw Honey –organic (optional)
- 2 tbsp. Water

Directions

1. Combine matcha tea, cinnamon and 2 tbsp. of water until mixed

2. Heat the coconut milk in a saucepan until warm

3. Pour the hot coconut milk mixture and tea in a blender to mix until well-combined

4. Pour the contents into a mug and sprinkle with a dash of matcha tea

5. Serve immediately and enjoy!

LUNCH: GROUNDED SWEET POTATOES AND SPINACH

Makes 2 Servings

Ingredients

- 4 Sweet Potatoes
- 2 Red apples – organic
- 2 cups Mushrooms
- 1¼ cups baby spinach
- 2 tsp. coconut oil –organic
- Salt and pepper

Directions

1. Peel and slice the sweet potatoes and apples into cubes

2. Cut mushrooms into strips

3. In a wok or a skillet, add the coconut oil to a medium heat

4. Stir in the sweet potatoes and cook for about 8 minutes

5. Add the remaining ingredients

6. Stir for another 5 minutes

7. Add salt and pepper, to taste

8. Serve immediately and enjoy!

SNACKS: SUPER ENERGETIC DRINK
Makes 1 Serving

Ingredients

- 2 apples – organic
- 1/2 cup raspberries
- 1 lemon - freshly squeezed
- 1 tbsp. Raw Honey –organic
- 1 tsp. acerola powder
- 1 tbsp. chia seeds

Directions

1. Rinse apples and cut into 4 pieces
2. Rinse raspberries
3. Place both ingredients into the juicer
4. Squeeze the lemon juice and add to the fruit mixture
5. Add honey, acerola powder and mix
6. Top with chia seeds and pour into a bottle
7. Place in the fridge and let cool
8. Serve cold and enjoy!

DINNER: GRILLED PORK CHOP
Makes 2 Servings

Ingredients

- 2 Pork chops
- 1 tbsp. olive oil – extra virgin
- 1 tbsp. lemon juice
- 1 tsp. of Honey – organic
- 1 tsp. Rosemary
- 1 tsp. Oregano
- Salt & Pepper

Directions

1. Mix the spices with the olive oil, honey, and lemon juice
2. Add the pork chops and marinate the mixture for 30 minutes, at least
3. Heat the grill and fry the pork chops
4. Cook until preference – around 7 minutes per side
5. Serve immediately and enjoy!

DAY 6

BREAKFAST: PALEO TORTILLA
Makes 2 Servings

Ingredients

- 1 Onion - chopped
- 1 Red Bell Pepper – stripped
- 2 Mushrooms of your choice - chopped
- 4 Eggs –beaten
- 1 tbsp. Olive oil
- Salt

Directions

1. In a skillet, add olive oil over low heat

2. Add the onions, bell pepper, and mushrooms and cook over low heat for 3 minutes

3. Add the eggs and cook for 1 minute on each side

4. Serve immediately and enjoy!

LUNCH: SCALLOPS WITH ZUCCHINI & CARROTS

Makes 2 Servings

Ingredients

- 6 scallops
- 1 orange carrot
- 1 yellow carrot
- ½ zucchini
- 1 tbsp. coconut oil

Directions

1. Clean and peel the carrots and zucchini

2. Use a peeling knife to shred the zucchini and carrots

3. Boil hot water and add the carrots and zucchini to cook for approximately 5 minutes

4. In a skillet, sauté coconut oil and scallops

5. Add the scallops, zucchini and carrots to your plate

6. Serve immediately and enjoy!

SNACK: STRAWBERRY SORBET
Makes 1 Serving

Ingredients

- 1 cup strawberries
- 1/4 cup apple juice – organic

Directions

1. Place the frozen strawberries in a mixer

2. Add the apple juice and blend on high

3. Continue until you achieve a smooth mixture

4. Serve immediately and enjoy!

DINNER: CHICKEN CURRY STIR FRIED PUMPKIN & SMOKED ALMOND

Makes 2 Servings

Ingredients

- 3 Chicken Breast fillets
- ½ pumpkin
- 1 shallot – chopped
- 1/3 cup coconut cream
- 4 tbsp. fish sauce
- Curry powder
- 1 oz. smoked almond
- 2 tbsp. coconut oil
- 2 tbsp. Olive oil
- Salt and Pepper
- Grated coconut
- A few Fresh chives

Directions

1. Cut the chicken breast into cubes and refrigerate for 10-20 minutes

2. Remove the seeds from the squash and cut into cubes – refrigerate

3. Chop the fresh chives finely – then refrigerate

4. Chop the shallot and almonds and set aside

5. Add olive oil to the skillet over high heat

6. Stir fry the squash

7. Add the almonds, salt, and pepper in the skillet

8. Add an additional 2 tbsp. of coconut oil and stir in the shallot

9. Once the shallot is golden brown, add the chicken until cooked

10. Stir in the curry powder and fish sauce to taste

11. Continue cooking for 1 minute and reduce until fish sauce is evaporated

12. Pour coconut cream and reduce to low heat until you achieve a creamy sauce

13. Garnish with grated coconut and chives

14. Serve immediately and enjoy!

DAY 7

BREAKFAST: RED FRUITS CRUMBLE
Makes 2 Servings

Ingredients

- 3 cups of red fruits - strawberries, raspberries, blackberries, blackcurrants
- 1 tbsp. vanilla powder
- 1 tbsp. cinnamon
- 2 tbsp. brown sugar
- 2/3 cup muesli - organic
- 2 tbsp. slivered almonds

Directions

1. Combine and mix the berries
2. Add vanilla powder, cinnamon, and brown sugar and mix
3. Pour the berry mixture into a baking dish
4. Top with almonds and organic muesli
5. Bake 25 minutes at 350 degrees F
6. Let it cool
7. Serve and enjoy!

LUNCH: STEAK TARTARE
Makes 1 Serving

Ingredients

- 8 oz. Beef butcher
- 1 egg – whole
- 2 shallots
- 2 tbsp. mustard
- 2 tbsp. olive oil
- Salt
- Pepper

Directions

1. Combine shallots, olive oil, mustard, vinegar, salt, and pepper to create a marinade
2. Add beef and combine with the marinade
3. Break an egg and put the egg yolk on the tartare.
4. Serve immediately and enjoy!

SNACK: SWEET POTATO CHIPS
Makes 1-2 Servings

Ingredients

- 2 sweet potatoes
- 1 tsp. salt
- 1 tsp. paprika
- 3 tbsp. olive oil

Directions

1. Wash and peel the sweet potatoes
2. Use a mandolin to cut thin slices
3. Place the sliced sweet potatoes in a plastic freezer bag
4. Add olive oil, salt and paprika
5. Mix the ingredients and place them over a baking sheet
6. Bake at the lowest heat settings for 3 hours or until golden brown
7. Serve and enjoy!

DINNER: SHRIMPS SKEWER WITH CITRUS SALAD

Makes 2 Servings

Ingredients

- 2 cups Shrimp
- 2 oranges – medium
- 1 lettuce head – chopped
- 1 grapefruit
- 1 mango - cubed
- 1 lemon
- 3 cherry tomatoes
- 1 tbsp. Balsamic Vinegar

Directions

For the Shrimps Skewer:

1. De-shell the shrimp and set aside
2. Peel the grapefruit and oranges and side ¼ aside for the salad
3. In a saucepan, add 4 tbsp. of olive oil over medium heat
4. Add the oranges and grapefruit and reduce to low heat
5. Cook for 15 minutes then add balsamic vinegar

6. Place the shrimp on pikes and season with salt and pepper to taste

7. Add olive oil to the pan and cook the shrimp

For the Citrus Salad:

1. Combine the mango, oranges, grapefruit, lettuce and cherry tomatoes

2. Drizzle the salad with olive oil

To Complete the Dish:

1. Set your salad and skewers on your plate

2. Serve immediately and enjoy!

WEEK 2
BREAKFAST OPTIONS

★ Tropical banana

★ 3 P's Green Smoothie

★ Egg & Avocado Cocotte

★ Paleo Eggs & Bacon

★ Pancakes Au Potiron

★ Paleo bacon & eggs

★ Pumpkin-Berry Smoothie

LUNCH OPTIONS

★ Salmon Tartare

★ Zucchini Spaghetti with Avocado Pesto

★ Orange Chicken Thighs

★ Back of Cod with thyme and small vegetables

★ Beet Salad with Pecans

★ Sea bass with herbs in a bag

★ Cod with little vegetables and lemon en papillote

SNACKS OPTIONS

★   Potimaron & Coco Biscuit

★   Energy balls

★   Vanilla Pumpkin Seed Clusters

★   Baked Kale Chips

★   Baked apples with Dates & Almond powder

★   Baked Cinnamon Apple Chips

★   Celtic Blueberry Muffins

DINNER OPTIONS

★   Roast Chicken with Herbs

★   Breaded Fish with Coconut with Avocado & Orange Salad

★   Paleo Chicken Burger

★   Italian meatballs

★   Paleo Lasagna

★   Zucchini & Shrimp Curry

★   Creamy Lemon Chicken with Asparagus and Mushrooms

Day 1

BREAKFAST: TROPICAL BANANA
Makes 1 Serving

Ingredients

- Banana – ripened
- 1 tsp. Coconut Oil – organic
- 1 tbsp. Grated Coconut –sweetened
- 1 tsp. Raw Honey –organic

Directions

1. Add coconut oil to a pan on low heat

2. Cut banana in half crosswise, then cut each piece in half lengthwise – resulting in 4 pieces

3. Cook the banana covered – about 2 minutes per side.

4. Sprinkle with grated coconut and add honey.

5. Serve warm and enjoy!

LUNCH: SALMON TARTARE
Makes 2 Servings

Ingredients

- 1/3 cup Smoked Salmon
- 7 oz. Fresh salmon
- 1 Lime – freshly squeezed
- 3 Cucumbers - diced
- 1 Shallot – chopped
- 2 tbsp. Paleo Mayonnaise
- 1 tbsp. Capers
- 1 tbsp. Chopped dill
- Salt and pepper

Directions

1. Chop the salmon in fine cuts
2. Add the lime squeeze and mix to combine
3. Dice the cucumbers and chop the shallot
4. Combine dill, capers, shallots, pickles, and mayonnaise with the salmon
5. Add salt and pepper, to taste.
6. Serve immediately and enjoy!

SNACK: POTIMARON & COCO BISCUIT
Makes 12 Servings

Ingredients

- 2/3 cup pumpkin
- 4 ounces almond puree
- 2 ounces of coconut sugar
- 1 egg
- 1/2 tsp. cinnamon
- 2 ounces almond flour
- 1 ounce of coconut flour
- 1.7 ounce of dark chocolate chips

Directions

1. Cook the pumpkin with steam for 20 minutes.
2. Mix the pumpkin puree with coconut sugar, almond flour, egg, and cinnamon.
3. Preheat oven to 350 ° F
4. Add the almond flour and coconut flour to the preceding mixture. Mix.
5. Add the chocolate chips and mix again.
6. Shape the cookies that you put on a baking sheet.
7. Bake for 15 minutes. Let cool before serving.
8. Serve immediately and enjoy!

DINNER: ROAST CHICKEN WITH HERBS
Makes 3 Servings

Ingredients

- 1 Whole Chicken – free-range, organic
- 8 potatoes
- 1 bunch Tarragon - fresh
- 1 bunch Basil – fresh
- 4 tbsp. olive oil
- Salt and pepper

Directions

1. Preheat oven to 350 ° F
2. Clean the chicken and put herbs inside.
3. Wash potatoes and cut each into 4 pieces – with skins on
4. Place the chicken in a dish and arrange the potatoes around the chicken
5. Drizzle with olive oil.
6. Bake for 1.5 hours, basting the chicken and potatoes with the juice every 30 minutes
7. Serve warm and enjoy!

DAY 2

BREAKFAST: 3 P'S GREEN SMOOTHIE
Makes 2 Servings

Ingredients

- 2 bananas – medium, ripened
- 1 Pear –organic
- 1 Apple - organic
- ½ bunch Parsley
- ¼ Avocado – ripened
- ½ Plum – medium
- ¼ cup water
- ¼ cup ice

Directions

1. Remove seed from plum, skin & seed from avocado, skin from bananas and stalks from pears and apples.
2. Chop all fruits into uniform size
3. Add the ingredients to blender and blend until smooth and creamy results
4. Serve immediately and enjoy!

LUNCH ZUCCHINI SPAGHETTI WITH AVOCADO PESTO

Makes 4 Servings

Ingredients

For the Spaghetti:

- 4 medium zucchini
- ½ cup cherry tomatoes - halved
- 1 Lemon or lime – freshly chopped
- Salt and pepper, to taste

For the Pesto:

¥ ¼ cup Pine nuts
¥ 1 Avocado – ripened
¥ 2 oz. Lemon juice – freshly squeezed
¥ 2 oz. Olive oil
¥ 2 Garlic cloves
¥ 1 bunch of Basil leaves – chopped

Directions

For the Spaghetti:

1. Peel the skin zucchini
2. With a vegetable grater, cut the zucchini to achieve spaghetti-like results

3. In a bowl, combine the zucchini spaghetti and cherry tomatoes with the pesto
4. Sprinkle with grated lemon zest
5. Add Salt and pepper, to taste

For the Pesto:

1. Heat a frying pan and toast the pine nuts until browned
2. Allow to cool on a plate
3. Meanwhile, add all ingredients in a blender and blend until smooth results
4. Adjust seasoning to taste
5. Add garlic, olive oil or lemon, if necessary
6. Serve immediately and enjoy!

**Be sure to store in the refrigerator up to 4 days.

SNACK: ENERGY BALLS
Makes 8 Servings

Ingredients

- 2/3 cup Dried Apricots
- 2/3 cup Ground Almonds
- 4 tbsp. water
- 2 tbsp. Raw Honey - organic
- Grated coconut
- Sesame seeds

Directions

1. Cut the apricots in half and place them in a blender

2. Add the remaining ingredients and blend until smooth

3. Roll the mixture into small balls and place them on a plate

4. Place the balls in the refrigerator and let chill for 15 minutes.

5. Roll the balls and cover in grated coconut and sesame seeds.

6. Serve immediately and enjoy!

DINNER: BREADED FISH WITH COCONUT WITH AVOCADO & ORANGE SALAD

Makes 4 Servings

Ingredients

For the Salad:

- 2 avocados
- 4 untreated oranges
- 1/2 cup dried grapes
- 2 tbsp. walnut oil
- 1 tsp. lemon juice
- 1 tbsp. sesame seeds
- 1 tsp. honey
- 2 pinches pepper
- Sea salt

For the fish:

- 4 cod fillets
- 3 eggs
- 1 tsp. ground coriander
- 1/2 cup of coconut flour
- 1/2 cup grated coconut
- Olive oil (for cooking)

Directions

For the salad:

1. Grill the sesame seeds in a dry pan for 2 minutes
2. Grate the zest of an orange and the press to collect the juice
3. Pour the juice into a bowl with honey, lemon juice, and pepper
4. Cut the remaining 3 oranges and avocados into pieces once peeled
5. Make your plates mixed with avocados and orange pieces
6. Drizzle the plate with a sauce of orange juice, then add the oil.
7. Garnish the dish with orange peels, raisins, toasted sesame seeds and salt.

For the Fish:

1. In a dish, beat eggs.
2. Add a tablespoon of coriander powder and a pinch of salt and pepper.
3. In a second plate, pour the coconut flour.
4. In a third plate, add the grated coconut.
5. Dip fish in coconut flour until completely covered.
6. Brush the fish with the egg mixture
7. Then add the fish in the grated coconut.
8. Add oil and heat the pan
9. Place the fish and brown on all sides.
10. Serve immediately and enjoy!

DAY 3

BREAKFAST: EGG & AVOCADO COCOTTE
Makes 2 Servings

Ingredients

- 2 eggs – whole, organic
- 1 avocado – ripened
- 1 garlic clove – chopped
- 1 tsp. Red pepper
- Salt and Pepper

Directions

1. Preheat oven to 425 F

2. Cut the avocado in half and remove the pits

3. Peel and chop the garlic

4. Rub the flesh on the inside of the avocado.

5. Crack the egg into the hollow of each half cut avocado.

6. Season with the red pepper, salt, and pepper.

7. Bake for 15 minutes

8. Serve immediately and enjoy!

LUNCH: ORANGE CHICKEN THIGHS
Makes 4 Servings

Ingredients

- 4 Chicken Thighs
- 1 Orange
- 2 Garlic cloves - crushed
- 2 tbsp. Olive oil
- 2 tbsp. Raw Honey – organic
- Juice of 2 Oranges – freshly squeezed
- 2 tsp. Orange Blossom water
- Salt and pepper, to taste

Directions

1. Combine all the ingredients except the chicken thighs in a bowl

2. Add the chicken thighs, wrap with cellophane

3. Let the chicken marinate set for 1 hour in the refrigerator

4. Preheat oven to 400 ° F

5. Cut the orange into thick slices and place one slice on each chicken thigh.

6. Place the orange chicken and bake for 20 minutes

7. Baste the chicken with the marine every 5 to 10 minutes, depending on your preference.

8. Serve immediately and enjoy!

SNACK: VANILLA PUMPKIN SEED CLUSTERS
Makes 2 Servings

Ingredients

- 1/2 cup pumpkin seeds
- 2 tsp. honey
- 2 tsp. coconut sugar
- 1 tsp. vanilla extract
- Water (previously boiled)

Directions

1. Preheat oven to 300 F.

2. In a medium bowl, combine the honey, coconut sugar and vanilla.

3. Stir to create a thick paste then add a small drop of boiled water to thin it out for smooth syrup

4. Pour in the pumpkin seeds and stir them around in the mixture to coat evenly.

5. Add a generous tsp. full of the pumpkin seeds onto a baking sheet

6. Repeat until it's all used up and cook for 15-20 minutes until most of the seeds have browned

7. Take out of the oven and leave to cool for a few minutes.

8. Once they've cooled a little you can press the clusters together to make sure they don't fall apart.

9. Serve and topping or as a cereal and enjoy!

DINNER: PALEO CHICKEN BURGER
Makes 2 Servings

Ingredients

- 2 Paleo Burger buns
- 1 Avocado
- 1 Chicken Breast – grilled
- 1 large handful of Lettuce leaves
- 1/2 cup grated Red Cabbage
- 2 tbsp. Guacamole
- Salt and pepper, to taste

Directions

1. Once you have grilled your chicken breast, place it on the burger buns
2. Add guacamole, red cabbage, lettuce leaves and avocado as toppings
3. Sprinkle with salt and pepper to taste
4. Serve immediately and enjoy!

DAY 4

BREAKFAST: PALEO EGGS & BACON
Makes 3 Servings

Ingredients

- 6 slices bacon - uncooked
- 6 eggs – fresh, whole
- Chives
- Salt and pepper

Directions

1. Preheat oven to 400 F

2. Place bacon slices in muffin tins,

3. Then break an egg on each tin.

4. Sprinkle with chopped chives, salt, and pepper.

5. Place in the oven and bake for ten minutes.

6. Remove each bacon cup and serve with seasonal vegetables or a green salad

7. Serve immediately and enjoy!

LUNCH: BACK OF COD WITH THYME AND SMALL VEGETABLES

Makes 2 Servings

Ingredients

- 1 cod fillet – about 14 oz.
- 2 leeks
- 2 carrots
- 4 sweet potatoes
- 5 thyme leaves
- 1 Lemon
- 1 handful of Herbs
- Salt and pepper

Directions

1. Peel and cut into strips the sweet potatoes

2. Cook them in the steamer for 10 minutes.

3. Meanwhile, peel the carrots and leeks and cut into thin strips.

4. Add them to cook with the sweet potatoes, and cook 5 more minutes.

5. Gently put the cod fillet on top of the vegetables with thyme leaves, herbs, lemon, salt, pepper.

6. Cook the dish for another 10 minutes

7. Serve immediately and enjoy!

SNACKS: BAKED KALE CHIPS
Makes 1-2 Servings

Ingredients

- 1 Head of Kale - washed thoroughly and dried
- 2 tbsp. Olive oil
- Sea salt, for flavor

Directions

1. Preheat oven to 350 degrees F

2. Remove the ribs of the kale and cut into 2-inch pieces

3. Place kale on a baking sheet, drizzle with olive oil, and sprinkle with sea salt

4. Bake the kale chips for 10-15 minutes until crisp, be sure to turn the leaves every few minutes

5. Remove from oven, let it cool

6. Serve warm or cool and enjoy!

DINNER: ITALIAN MEATBALLS
Makes 4 Servings

Ingredients

For the meat balls

- 3 1/3 cups of chopped Steak
- 1 Egg - lightly beaten
- ½ Onion – chopped
- 2 Cloves Garlic - crushed
- 2 tbsp. Ground Almonds
- 1 tbsp. chopped Parsley
- 4 tbsp. Tomato paste
- 1 tbsp. Olive oil
- ½ cup vegetable broth
- Chopped basil

For the tomato sauce

- 2 ½ cups of crushed Tomatoes
- 1 Garlic clove - crushed
- 4 tbsp. dried tomato paste
- 1 tbsp. Olive oil

Directions

To Prepare to Meat balls:

1. In a bowl, mix the minced meat, onion, garlic, almonds and egg by hand
2. Add the parsley and half the tomato paste and mix
3. Form twenty balls – about the size of a ping pong ball

To cook the Tomato sauce:

1. In a pan over medium heat, stir-fry the garlic for a few minutes in olive oil,
2. Add the chopped onions and dried tomato paste and stir constantly.
3. Simmer for 15 minutes

To cook the Meat balls:

1. Heat the remaining tablespoon olive oil over high heat in a frying pan
2. Add in the meat balls and cook for 1 min approx. - turning them with a wooden spoon.
3. Add the tomato sauce, vegetable broth, and the remaining tomato paste.
4. Reduce heat and cook 10 minutes covered with lid
5. Reduce the heat and cook 5 more minutes without the lid.
6. Sprinkle with parsley and basil and serve hot.
7. Serve immediately and enjoy!

DAY 5

BREAKFAST: PANCAKES AU POTIRON
Makes 2 Servings

Ingredients

- 2 oz. of mashed Pumpkin
- 2 tbsp. of Almond milk
- 2 eggs – fresh, whole
- 1/2 cup of almond flour
- 1 tsp. of Maple syrup
- 1 tbsp. Vanilla extract
- 2 tbsp. Coconut flour
- 2 tsp. of vegetable oil
- ½ tsp. baking soda
- ½ tsp. ground Cinnamon
- 1 pinch ground Ginger
- 1 pinch of salt
- 1 pinch of ground Cloves

Directions

1. In a bowl, mix the pumpkin puree, eggs, almond milk, maple syrup and vanilla extract until creamy.
2. In another bowl, combine coconut flour, baking soda, salt, almond flour, cinnamon, ginger and cloves.

3. Pour the pumpkin and flour mixture in a container with a spout and mix until well combined

4. Heat vegetable oil in a pan over low heat and pour several small ladles of batter into the hot oil to form rounded pancakes

5. Cook until pancakes are lightly browned, about 5 minutes per side.

6. Serve immediately and enjoy!

LUNCH: BEET SALAD WITH PECANS
Makes 4 Servings

Ingredients

- 1 cup Lettuce – chopped
- 3 Beetroots - cooked
- ½ cup Pecans
- 1 large Shallot
- 3 tbsp. Soy cream
- 1 tbsp. Walnut oil
- Salt and pepper

Directions

1. Wash the lettuce and chop into salad slices
2. Chop the shallot and the pecans.
3. Cut the beetroot into thin slices, using a mandolin.
4. Mix the soy cream, walnut oil, salt and pepper in a bowl until well-combined.
5. Place lettuce, beetroot, pecans and shallot in the plates
6. Season according to taste
7. Serve immediately and enjoy!

SNACK: BAKED APPLES WITH DATES & ALMOND POWDER

Makes 2 Servings

Ingredients

- 2 apples – organic
- 4 dates
- 1 tbsp. of almond powder

Directions

1. Preheat the oven to 350 F
2. Wash apples and remove the core
3. Mix the chopped dates and almonds
4. Fill the almond mix inside the apples.
5. Bake for 30 minutes, allow to cool
6. Serve warm and enjoy!

DINNER: PALEO LASAGNA
Makes 2 Servings

Ingredients

For the meat & tomato sauce:

- 18 oz. minced Beef
- 18 oz. Tomatoes - about 5 medium-sized
- 2 Onions - chopped
- 1 Garlic clove
- Tomato puree
- Oregano
- Salt

For the Paleo "white sauce":

- 3.5 oz. walnuts
- 1.7 oz. almonds
- 6.7 oz. Water

For the "pasta lasagna":

- 1 cup eggplant - about 2 medium-sized

Directions

1. Cut the eggplant slices for about ¼ -inch - if the slices are too thin, they will burn in the oven.

2. Using a brush, brush the slices with olive oil eggplant

3. Bake at 325 F in grill mode for about 10 minutes

4. Once the eggplant slices begin to brown, flip the slices.

5. Cut the onion and garlic and fry on the skillet in olive oil until onions are translucent

6. Prepare the ground beef by forming small balls by hand

7. Add them to the pan with the onions and stir

8. Cut the tomatoes into slices and add them to the pan when the meat is cooked on the surface and continue to stir

9. Mix the walnuts, almonds and water together and combine

10. You will get a dough which should be the consistency of a thick sauce, not liquid.

11. If it is too mushy, add water. You must be able to spread easily.

12. Pour half of the water and add the tomato paste to give consistency.

13. Adjust seasoning with salt and oregano, and stir.

14. Pour 1/3 of the beef-onion-tomato mixture into the baking dish

15. Cover with a layer of eggplant slices, then your walnut-almond preparation.

16. Repeat step 8 until complete

17. Finish by covering your beef-onion-tomato preparation.

18. Be sure not to finish with the walnut-almond mixture.

19. Bake 20 minutes at 325 F

20. Serve immediately and enjoy!

DAY 6

BREAKFAST: PALEO BACON AND EGGS
Makes 1 Serving

Ingredients

- 3 Eggs - whole
- 2 Bacon slices
- 1 tbsp. Olive oil
- 1 tbsp. Pesto
- 1 tbsp. Tapenade

Directions

1. Gently place 2 eggs in a pot of boiling water.

2. Remove the first egg after 3 minutes – soft-boiled egg

3. Remove the second egg after 10 minutes – hard-boiled egg.

4. Cook the bacon in a skillet until crispy.

5. Break an egg into a bowl and mix it with tapenade and pesto.

6. Cook the mixture to the skillet

7. Serve immediately and enjoy!

LUNCH: SEA BASS WITH HERBS IN A BAG
Makes 2 Servings

Ingredients

- 500g of Sea Bass
- 3 Tomatoes - medium
- 1 Lemon
- 2 tbsp. Olive oil
- ½ cup Dry White Wine - optional
- Thyme
- Basil
- 3 Garlic cloves

Directions

1. Preheat oven to 400 F
2. Remove guts from the Sea bass and clean
3. Place your herbs, olive oil and white wine (optional) inside.
4. Place the Sea Bass in aluminum foil and seal
5. Cut the tomatoes in half and place on bottom of the dish.
6. Season the tomatoes and place the Sea Bass in its aluminum foil on top.
7. Cook in the oven for 40 minutes
8. Serve immediately and enjoy!

SNACK: BAKED CINNAMON APPLE CHIPS
Makes 1-2 Servings

Ingredients

- 1-2 apples – organic (I used Honeycrisp)
- 1 tsp. cinnamon

Directions

1. Preheat oven to 395 °F

2. Remove seeds, then slice apples thinly - using a sharp knife or mandolin

3. Prepare a baking sheet with parchment paper and arrange apple slices – be sure not to overlap Sprinkle cinnamon over apples.

4. Bake for 1 hour, then flip.

5. Continue baking for 1-2 hours more, flipping occasionally - until the apple slices are no longer moist.

6. Serve immediately and enjoy!

*Store in airtight container when not consuming

DINNER: ZUCCHINI & SHRIMP CURRY
Makes 2 Servings

Ingredients

- 6 pieces of shrimp
- 1 zucchini – large
- 1 red onion - chopped
- 1 can of Coconut milk – organic
- 2 tsp. Red Curry paste
- 1 tsp. Coconut oil – organic

Directions

1. Chop the onion and cut the zucchini into diced pieces

2. In a wok or frying pan, melt the coconut oil.

3. Fry the onion, then add the coconut milk and curry paste.

4. Once the curry paste is well-dissolved, add the zucchini.

5. Allow to simmer for 2-3 minutes then add the shrimp.

6. Simmer for another 10 minutes

7. Serve immediately and enjoy!

DAY 7

BREAKFAST: EGGS BENEDICT WITH CREAMY AVOCADO SAUCE
Makes 4 Servings

Ingredients

- 5 strips of bacon - cut into half pieces
- 4 eggs - whole
- Sea salt
- Freshly ground black pepper

For the avocado sauce:

- 1 medium avocado, peeled
- 1/4 cup lemon juice
- 1/2 tsp. garlic powder
- 1/3 cup olive oil or water
- Sea salt

Directions

1. Preheat your oven to 400 F.

2. On a baking sheet, arrange the bacon into four separate bases for the eggs

3. Each base should be a few pieces of bacon arranged in a weave pattern

4. Cook the bacon bases in the oven for 15 to 20 minutes.

5. Puree the avocado, lemon juice and garlic powder in a food processor until smooth.

6. Add the olive oil or water until you get a thick, pourable consistency.

7. Season to taste with sea salt

8. Bring a pot of water to a boil, drop an egg in, and let it cook until the whites are set, about 2-4 minutes

9. Remove and repeat with the remaining eggs.

10. Divide the bacon among the plates, top with the poached eggs

11. Pour avocado sauce on top of each egg.

12. Serve immediately and enjoy!

LUNCH: COD WITH LITTLE VEGETABLES AND LEMON EN PAPILLOTE
Makes 4 Servings

Ingredients

- 4 Cod fillets
- 2 cups of green peas, baby carrots and green beans mix
- 2 Garlic clove
- 1 tbsp. Raw Honey – organic
- 1 tbsp. Olive oil
- Dill – chopped, fresh
- Lime wedge
- Juice of 1 Lime – fresh squeezed
- Juice of 1 Lemon – freshly squeezed
- Salt and pepper

Directions

1. Mix lemon juice, honey and olive oil in a bowl.

2. Marinate cod fillets in the mixture for 1 hour.

3. Clean the vegetables, pod the peas, and hull the green beans.

4. Peel and cut the carrots into small cubes.

5. Peel and chop the garlic.

6. In four large sheets of aluminum foil, spread the vegetables, garlic and cod fillets on top.

7. Sprinkle with Salt and pepper to taste

8. Drizzle with olive oil and lime juice.

9. Seal the aluminum foil and cook on the barbecue for 20-30 minutes.

10. Sprinkle with chopped dill and served immediately with fresh lemon wedges.

11. Enjoy!

SNACK: CELTIC BLUEBERRY MUFFINS
Makes 12 Servings

Ingredients

- 3 large Eggs
- 2 cups blanched almond flour
- 1 cup blueberries – fresh
- ½ cup tapioca flour
- 1/3 cup Raw Honey - organic
- ¼ cup virgin coconut oil, ghee or pastured butter – melted
- ½ teaspoon Baking soda
- ½ teaspoon Baking powder - gluten-free
- ½ teaspoon sea salt
- 1 teaspoon vanilla extract

Directions

1. Preheat the oven to 325 degrees F.
2. Grease a regular sized muffin tin or line with paper liners. *You can also use a silicone pan or silicone cupcake liners for better "non-stick" results
3. Mix (or sift) the dry ingredients together in a medium bowl.
4. Whisk the eggs, honey, oil and vanilla in another bowl.
5. Pour the wet ingredients into the bowl with the dry ingredients and stir until well combined.
6. Gently stir the blueberries into the batter.
7. Spoon into 12 muffin tins.
8. Bake for 20-25 minutes until slightly golden on top.
9. Serve warm and enjoy!

DINNER: CREAMY LEMON CHICKEN WITH ASPARAGUS AND MUSHROOMS
Makes 4 Servings

Ingredients

- 3-4 large chicken breasts
- 8 asparagus spears - medium-sized cut into 1 inch pieces
- 8 oz. sliced mushrooms
- 2 tbsp. coconut oil
- 3 garlic cloves - crushed
- ¾ cup coconut milk –organic
- Juice of 1 lemon – freshly squeezed
- Zest of 1 lemon
- Salt, to taste

Directions

1. Begin by heating up a large skillet to medium - high heat.
2. Once hot, add 1 tbsp. coconut oil.
3. Place chicken in pan, heat about 3 minutes per side, and set aside
4. Add remaining coconut oil, if needed.
5. Toss in crushed garlic, asparagus, and mushrooms.

6. Sauté until asparagus is crispy, and mushrooms are soft and fragrant - about 10 minutes

7. Return the chicken to the pan.

8. Add in coconut milk, lemon juice, and lemon zest.

9. With the skillet over medium-high heat, and cover.

10. Wait until the mixture bubbles, then reduce medium-low heat.

11. Cook for an additional 3-5 minutes or until the chicken is cooked through.

12. Add salt to taste and serve with rice, pasta, or zoodles.

13. Serve immediately and enjoy!

WEEK 3
BREAKFAST OPTIONS

★ Chia & red berries pudding

★ Prosciutto Eggs

★ Coco Flakes

★ Vegetable Omelet

★ Plantain Tortilla

★ Gruau Paleo Surprise

★ Pumpkin-Berry Smoothie

LUNCH OPTIONS

★ Paleo Squash with Walnuts

★ Paleo Pork Wrap

★ Cucumber & Mint Greek Salad

★ Black Olives Tapenade

★ Rolled Spinach & Goat

★ Thai beef salad

★ Crispy Shrimp with Coconut

SNACK OPTIONS

- ★ Chocolate Energy "Shot Blocks"
- ★ Paleo Energy Bars
- ★ Toasted pumpkin seeds with spices
- ★ Coconut Lemon Energy Balls
- ★ Nutty Fruit Balls
- ★ Carrot & Cardamom Bites
- ★ Curried Cashews

DINNER OPTIONS

- ★ Basil beef & green peppers wok
- ★ India-style chicken
- ★ Sea Stew
- ★ Chicken Stew with Apples and Plums
- ★ Pizza Paleo
- ★ Cod and vegetables papillote with green lemon
- ★ Fish & Grapes Salad

DAY 1

BREAKFAST: CHIA & RED BERRIES PUDDING
Makes 2 Servings

Ingredients

- 7 oz. of Almond milk
- 3 tbsp. of Chia seeds
- 2 tbsp. of Coconut Sugar
- 1 pinch of vanilla powder
- 1 large handful red berries - fresh or frozen

Directions

The night before:
1. Mix chia seeds, sugar, coconut and vanilla with the almond milk
2. Allow to chill and refrigerate overnight

The next morning:

1. Pour chia seeds in the pudding in 2 serving bowls
2. Top with red fruits
3. Sprinkle with crushed almonds on top – optional
4. Serve immediately and enjoy!

LUNCH: PALEO SQUASH WITH WALNUTS
Makes 2 Servings

Ingredients

- 2 tbsp. coconut oil
- 1 large yellow squash - grated
- 1 large tomato - cut into chunks
- ½ cup nuts
- 3 garlic cloves - chopped

Directions

1. Melt coconut oil in a skillet over medium heat

2. Add the grated yellow squash, tomato pieces, nuts and garlic, and cook in a pan.

3. Stir until the mixture is hot – about 3-5 minutes.

4. Serve immediately and enjoy!

SNACK: CHOCOLATE ENERGY "SHOT BLOCKS"

Makings about 15 Servings

Ingredients

- ⅔ cup of canned full-fat coconut milk - organic
- ⅔ cup of filtered water
- 2-4 Tbsp. Coconut Oil
- 2-3 Tbsp. Raw Honey or Maple Syrup - optional
- 3 Tbsp. Gelatin - grass-fed
- 3 Tbsp. Raw Cacao powder
- 2 Tbsp. Raw Maca powder
- 1 tsp. Vanilla extract
- ¼ tsp. Sea salt

Directions:

1. Combine all ingredients in a medium saucepan and whisk well.
2. Turn the heat to medium-low and cook until just warmed through to melt the gelatin -- do not boil.
3. Pour the mix into glass baking dish or molds of your choice.
4. Move it to the refrigerator to set for at least 1 hour.

5. Remove the blocks from the molds or the baking dish

6. Slice into desired size

7. Serve immediately and enjoy!

*Be sure to keep them in the refrigerator for up to a week.

DINNER: BASIL BEEF AND GREEN PEPPERS WOK
Makes 4 Servings

Ingredients

- 14oz. of Beef – sliced thinly
- 3 Green Peppers
- 1 tbsp. Olive oil – extra virgin
- 1 onion – chopped
- 1 bunch Basil –chopped thinly
- 1 garlic clove – sliced
- 1 tbsp. Arrowroot Powder (dissolved in 4 tbsp. water)

Directions

1. Slice the beef into thin slices and set apart

2. Wash the green peppers and cut into strips – remove the stalk and seeds

3. In a medium-sized wok, drizzle olive oil and place over medium heat

4. Prepare the onion and fry in wok until softened

5. Stir in the beef and peppers and cook until the meat is brown

6. Add the garlic clove

7. While the meat is cooking, slice the basil leaves thinly and add to the wok

8. Once the peppers soften, add the arrowroot powder mixture

9. Stir until you achieve a smooth texture

10. Remove wok from heat

11. Serve immediately and enjoy!

DAY 2

BREAKFAST: PROSCIUTTO EGGS
Makes 2 Servings

Ingredients

- Coconut oil – organic
- 4 slices prosciutto
- 4 eggs
- Salt, pepper and desired seasonings

Directions

1. Preheat the oven to 350F
2. Grease a muffin tin
3. Put your prosciutto slices to cover the bottom of the muffin.
4. Break an egg inside.
5. Season to taste.
6. Bake about 20 minutes for a creamy yellow result - 15 minutes for it to be flowing and 25 minutes for it to be cooked
7. Let cool and unmold.
8. Serve immediately and enjoy!

LUNCH: PALEO PORK WRAP
Makes 2 Servings

Ingredients

- 1 cup Pork tenderloin
- 2 tbsp. Homemade Paleo Mayonnaise
- 3 Cherry Tomatoes
- 1 Avocado
- 6 Lettuce leaves
- Vegetable oil
- Salt and pepper.

Directions

1. Place lettuce leaves on a plate.
2. Cut the pork into strips
3. Add oil to the pan and raise to a medium-heat
4. Fry the pork until cooked
5. Spread them in lettuce leaves with cherry tomatoes and avocado slices.
6. Season to your taste then roll the leaves to form wraps.
7. Serve immediately and enjoy!

SNACK: PALEO ENERGY BARS
Makes 1 Serving

Ingredients

- 20 dates
- 1 cup almonds
- 4 tbsp. coconut - grated

Directions

1. In a blender, add pitted dates, almonds and grated coconut.
2. Mix to obtain a paste-like result
3. Spread cellophane wrap and place the dough.
4. Close the paper and shape the dough to a brick
5. Allow to refrigerate overnight
6. Serve and enjoy!

DINNER: INDIA-STYLE CHICKEN
Makes 2 Servings

Ingredients

- 35oz. of chicken thighs
- 1 red onion, diced
- 2 cloves garlic, minced
- 1/2 cup coconut milk
- 4 tbsp. ghee
- 3 tbsp. coconut oil
- ¥ 1/2 tsp. cardamom
- ¥ 1/2 tsp. coriander
- ¥ 1 tsp. chili powder
- ¥ 1 can of tomato paste -12oz.
- ¥ 1 tsp. salt

Directions

1. Cut the thighs into portions of a bite-size

2. In a large skillet, heat oil coconut oil over medium heat.

3. Add onion and fry until transparent.

4. Lower the fire to a minimum and add the garlic and all the spices.

5. Mix well to form a kind of paste.

6. In a medium heat and add the coconut milk and salt.

7. Mix well to form a thick sauce.

8. When the sauce begins to bubble, add the chicken and mix well.

9. Reduce heat to medium-low, cover and cook for about 15 minutes - until the chicken is cooked

10. Stir occasionally

11. When the chicken is cooked, add the ghee and mix into the sauce until it melts.

12. Serve with vegetables of your choice.

13. Enjoy!

DAY 3

BREAKFAST: COCO FLAKES
Makes 2 Servings

Ingredients

- 1/2 cup coconut - flaked, unsweetened
- 1/2 cup berries - any
- 1/4 cup coconut milk
- Cinnamon
- 1 tsp. honey
- Nuts

Directions:

1. Toast the coconut flakes on medium-low heat in a pan.
2. Combine with red fruit choice
3. Pour the coconut milk and add cinnamon, honey and nuts
4. Mix until well-combined
5. Serve immediately and enjoy!

LUNCH: CUCUMBER & MINT GREEK SALAD

Makes 2 Servings

Ingredients

- 1 Cucumber - Organic
- ½ cup Coconut cream or Greek yogurt
- 1 tbsp. lemon juice – freshly squeezed
- Handful of Mint – fresh
- Handful of Parsley - fresh
- ½ Garlic clove – chopped
- Salt and pepper, to taste

Directions

1. Cut the cucumber into thin slices.

2. Sprinkle with salt and set aside in a bowl to make the sauce.

3. During this time it will discharge - part of the water from cucumber will be absorbed by the salt.

4. Chop the parsley and mint

5. Crush the garlic clove

6. Prepare the sauce by mixing the remaining ingredients

7. Put cucumbers to drain in a bowl

8. Add the sauce and mix well

9. Keep cool for 1 hour, until the flavors are spread well.

SNACK: TOASTED PUMPKIN SEEDS WITH SPICES

Makes 1 Serving

Ingredients

- 1 cup Pumpkin seeds
- 1 tbsp. Olive oil
- 1 tsp. of curry, turmeric, paprika, or cumin.
- ½ tsp. Salt

Directions

1. Rinse and dry the pumpkin seeds.

2. Preheat oven to 325 F and prepare a sheet of baking paper on a baking rack.

3. Mix all ingredients in a bowl so that all seeds are coated with oil and spices.

4. Spread them on the baking paper and bake for 40 minutes.

5. Watch the baking and occasionally stir the seeds to cook evenly.

6. Let cool slightly and enjoy them still warm or cold

DINNER: SEA STEW
Makes 4 Servings

Ingredients

- 2 cups fresh mussels - cleaned
- 1 cup Squid
- 2 cups cod fillets, or other white fish of choice
- 2 cups Tomatoes
- 1 Red pepper
- 1 Onion
- 2 cloves of Garlic
- 4 Bay leaves
- 1 fish stock cube - organic
- 1 tsp. of Turmeric and paprika
- 1 tsp. olive oil
- A few pinches salt and pepper

Directions

1. Cut the tomatoes and peppers into diced.

2. Finely chop the onion and garlic.

3. Heat the oil in a large pot

4. Add the onion and wait 2 minutes, then add garlic and spices.

5. Add the stock cube diluted in an 8 oz. glass of water

6. Then add the diced peppers and tomatoes and bay leaves.

7. Reduce to low heat and simmer for ten minutes.

8. Cut fish fillets into large cubes add them to the pot.

9. After two minutes, add the squid and mussels

10. Cover for 5 minutes and cook until the mussels are all open.

11. Stir gently and serve immediately

12. Enjoy!

DAY 4

BREAKFAST: VEGETABLE OMELET
Makes 1-2 Servings

Ingredients

- 1 cup cooked seasonal vegetables
- 3 eggs - whole
- 3 tbsp. coconut milk - organic
- 1 tsp. of coconut oil
- Salt and pepper

Directions

1. Melt the coconut oil in skillet over medium heat
2. Fry the vegetables in oil to warm
3. In a bowl, beat eggs with whisk with salt and pepper
4. Add the coconut milk and whisk again
5. Turn the stove on low heat
6. Spread the vegetables in the bottom of the pan and pour the egg and coconut milk mixture
7. Cover and cook for about 15 minutes
8. The frittata is cooked when it is no longer liquid on top
9. Serve immediately and enjoy!

LUNCH: BLACK OLIVES TAPENADE
Makes 2 Servings

Ingredients

- 2/3 cup Black olives
- 1/4 cup Anchovies
- 1/4 cup Capers - drained
- 1 Garlic clove
- 1/4 cup Olive oil
- Pepper

Directions

1. Place all the ingredients in a blender and mix until well blended
2. You can also add basil or spices of your choice.
3. If the tapenade is too dry, add a little olive oil.
4. Enjoy the spread on toasted Paleo bread
5. Serve immediately and enjoy!

SNACK: COCONUT LEMON ENERGY BALLS
Makes 18 Servings

Ingredients

- 1 Lemon, zest
- 2 Lemons, juice
- ¼ cup Chia seeds
- 1 ½ cup Raw almonds
- 8 dates - pitted & chopped
- ½ cup unsweetened shredded coconut (plus for more garnish, if desired)
- ¼ tsp. sea salt
- 3 tbsp. Coconut oil - organic

Directions

1. Zest 1 lemon and set it aside.
2. Juice 2 lemons into a small bowl.
3. Add the chia and mix well.
4. Combine almonds and dates in the bowl of a large food processor.
5. Process until finely ground, about 60 seconds.
6. Add shredded coconut, sea salt, coconut oil, zest, and chia/lemon juice mixture.

7. Process until the mixture is lumpy and moist, about 60 seconds.

8. Roll the mixture into 2" balls.   Sprinkle with coconut, if desired.

9. Refrigerate 30 minutes to set.

10. Serve and enjoy!

*Keep refrigerated in a sealed container.

DINNER: CHICKEN STEW WITH APPLES AND PLUMS
Makes 2 Servings

Ingredients

- 2 cups chicken breast
- 5 large carrots, cut into large pieces
- 1 1/2 large onion, cut into chunks
- 2 1/2 apples - cut into chunks
- 10 dried plums, pitted
- 1 coconut milk can
- 2 tsp. sea salt

For the filling:
- fresh sage, finely chopped

Directions

1 Cut the chicken breast into chunks and place in bottom of slow cooker.

2 Add the carrots, onions, apples and prunes.

3 Pour the coconut milk over all.

4 Simmer for 8 hours on low heat.

5 When cooked, mix all ingredients and season with salt to taste.

6 Serve with a sprinkling of fresh sage trim.

DAY 5

BREAKFAST: PLANTAIN TORTILLA
Makes 2 Servings

Ingredients

• 4 plantains

Directions

1. Preheat oven to 375 F
2. Cut plantains into 3 pieces, with peels
3. Boil 15 minutes until they are tender.
4. Drain and Cool, then remove the peels.
5. Crush coarsely
6. Train 6 tortillas with your hands and place on a baking sheet lined with parchment paper
7. Bake in oven 350 F for 15 minutes.
8. Turn and cook another 10 minutes.
9. Allow to cool for another 10 minutes
10. Serve warm and enjoy!

LUNCH: ROLLED SPINACH & GOAT
Makes 4 Servings

Ingredients

- 8 Eggs - whole
- 4 oz. of Spinach - fresh or frozen
- 7 oz. Fresh goat cheese
- 4 slices of Smoked salmon
- Handful of Parsley
- 1 Garlic clove
- Salt and pepper, to taste

Directions

1. Start by preheating the oven to 400 F

2. Mix parsley, garlic, spinach and eggs together.

3. Pour into a mold

4. Place in oven and bake 15-20 min.

5. Reduce the heat if you see that your omelet become brown.

6. Once the omelet is cooked, remove from mold.

7. Spread goat cheese and arrange the slices of smoked salmon.

8. Roll the omelet on itself and tighten using the plastic wrap.

9. Refrigerate the omelet to let it set and keep the shape.

10. Slice it into servings

11. Serve immediately and enjoy!

SNACKS: NUTTY FRUIT BALLS
Makes 12 Servings

Ingredients

- 2/3 cup mixed nuts - walnuts, cashews, hazelnuts, almonds, etc.
- 1 cup 1/2 of dates and/or figs
- 2 tsp. coconut oil
- 3 tbsp. Grated coconut
- Sunflower seeds, as toppings

Directions

1. Put all ingredients in a food processor

2. Blend until you obtain a dough

3. Empty the mixture into a bowl and add the sunflower seeds

4. Take a bit of dough in the palm of your hand to form a ball by packing well so it keeps its shape.

5. Store in the fridge for at least 1 hour

6. Serve chilled and enjoy!

*The balls can be stored in the fridge in an airtight container for several days.

DINNER: PIZZA PALEO
Makes 6 Servings

Ingredients

For the dough:

- 1/8 cup Coconut flour
- 2 oz. Almonds
- 4 eggs - large
- 4 tbsp. Olive oil
- 1 tsp. Baking soda
- 2 tbsp. Vinegar or lemon juice - to activate the baking soda
- Salt, pepper, oregano, and herbs, to taste

For the filling:

- 2 handfuls of Arugula
- 6 Parma ham slices
- Olives (black, green)

Directions

1. Preheat oven to 425 F

2. Mix all ingredients for the pizza dough.

3. Let the food processor or by hand.

4. If the consistency allows it, spread it thinly on a baking sheet with parchment paper or pour it into a dish

5. Spread it between 2 sheets of baking paper

6. Place in the oven and bake for 15 minutes or until dough is cooked.

7. Once the dough is golden, remove it from the oven and garnish it.

8. Add the tomato sauce base to moisten the dough, if it is too dry.

9. Bake for about 20 minutes.

10. Serve immediately and enjoy!

DAY 6

BREAKFAST: GRUAU PALEO SURPRISE
Makes 2 Servings

Ingredients

- 2-3 tbsp. Coconut oil
- 1 cup grated cauliflower
- 2 - 3 eggs, depending on size
- A handful of berries - fresh or frozen
- 2-3 tbsp. maple syrup or raw honey (optional)
- 2-3 tbsp. Coconut milk (optional)

Directions

1. Melt butter in a pan.

2. Add the grated cauliflower and the eggs.

3. Cook, stirring frequently as if you were making scrambled eggs.

4. Once the eggs are almost cooked, add the berries. Stir and heat for a few minutes.

5. Pour into a serving bowl topped with maple syrup and/or coconut milk.

LUNCH: THAI BEEF SALAD
Makes 2 Servings

Ingredients

- 2 (10 oz.) of Beef fillet
- 1 tbsp. Olive oil
- 1 handful chopped coriander + a few sprigs for presentation
- 1 handful mint - chopped
- 2 or 3 bird chilies - finely chopped
- 1 Garlic clove
- Juice of 1 lemon
- 2cm fresh ginger - grated
- 1 tbsp. of Raw Honey – organic
- 8 radish - sliced
- ½ cup cucumber - finely chopped
- 1 red onion - very thinly sliced
- Pepper, to taste

Directions

1. Put the meat in a nonstick frying pan with olive oil for 2 to 3 min per side.
2. Let stand 5 minutes on a hot plate.
3. In a bowl, mix herbs, peppers, garlic, lemon juice, ginger and honey.

4. Cut the beef into thin slices and put them in the marinade, while preparing the salad.

5. On a plate, add slices of radish, cucumber and onion,

6. Then add the meat, sauce and marinade

7. Finish seasoning with pepper

8. Sprinkle the dish with chopped coriander.

9. Serve immediately and enjoy!

SNACKS: CARROT & CARDAMOM BITES
Makes 1 Serving

Ingredients

- 2 ½ cups dried coconut –organic
- 1 cup carrots - steamed and cooled
- 1 tsp. powdered cardamom tea
- 1 tsp. powdered ginger

Directions

1. Place 2 cups of dried coconut in a food processor a few minutes to get a creamy texture.

2. Add the cooled cooked carrots and continue to mix to achieve puree results

3. Pour into a mixing bowl and add 1/2 cup of grated coconut

4. Stir until the flakes are well combined in the mixture.

5. Form 20-25 balls by rolling between your palms

6. Place them in the fridge and let it set for 1 hour

7. Serve chilled and enjoy!

DINER
COD WITH LITTLE VEGETABLES AND LEMON EN PAPILLOTE
Makes 4 Servings

Ingredients

- 4 Cod fillets
- 2 cups of green peas, baby carrots and green beans mix
- 2 Garlic clove
- 1 tbsp. Raw Honey – organic
- 1 tbsp. Olive oil
- Dill – chopped, fresh
- Lime wedge
- Juice of 1 Lime – fresh squeezed
- Juice of 1 Lemon – freshly squeezed
- Salt and pepper

Directions

1. Mix lemon juice, honey and olive oil in a bowl.

2. Marinate cod fillets in the mixture for 1 hour.

3. Clean the vegetables, pod the peas, and hull the green beans.

4. Peel and cut the carrots into small cubes.

5. Peel and chop the garlic.

6. In four large sheets of aluminum foil, spread the vegetables, garlic and cod fillets on top.

7. Sprinkle with Salt and pepper to taste

8. Drizzle with olive oil and lime juice.

9. Seal the aluminum foil and cook on the barbecue for 20-30 minutes.

10. Sprinkle with chopped dill and served immediately with fresh lemon wedges.

11. Enjoy!

DAY 7

BREAKFAST: PUMPKIN-BERRY SMOOTHIE
Makes 2 Servings

Ingredients

- 1 cup preferred non-dairy milk
- ½ cup fresh pumpkin puree
- ¼ cup cranberries – fresh or frozen
- ¼ cup raw cashews - soaked
- 1 small apple -chunked
- ½ orange, peeled
- 2 tablespoons coconut cream
- ¾ teaspoon cinnamon
- 5-10 drops Raw Honey – organic optional

Instructions

1. Place all ingredients in a high-powered blender and blend until smooth.

LUNCH: CRISPY SHRIMP WITH COCONUT
Makes 4 Servings

Ingredients

- 10 ounces prawns - peeled
- 3 tbsp. powdered coconut
- 4 tbsp. soup
- 2 tbsp. Olive oil
- Juice of 1 lemon or lime – freshly squeezed
- 1 handful of coriander - chopped
- Ground pepper - fresh

For the sauce:

- 6-8 tbsp. coconut milk soup
- 1 tbsp. sesame oil
- 1 tbsp. sesame seeds

For the Side Dish:

- 14 oz. broccoli
- 2 tbsp. almond or olive oil
- 2 tablespoons blanched almonds

Directions
1. Place the shrimp in a freezer bag with powdered coconut, and pepper

2. Stir several times to mix well over the shrimp.

For the sauce:

1. Heat a saucepan over low heat, and stir in all the ingredients, stir.

2. Simmer a few minutes, then pour into a bowl.

For the Side Dish:

1. Put a pan of water to boil and dip the broccoli florets for 3 to 4 minutes.

2. Drain and rinse them under cold water to stop the cooking and preserve the color green.

3. Put the broccoli in another bowl, sprinkled with almond oil (or olive oil)

4. Sprinkle with blanched almonds.

To Cook the Shrimp:

1. In a pan with the olive oil over medium heat

2. Fry the shrimp 3 to 4 min. stirring often.

3. Arrange them on a dish, seasoned with lemon juice

4. Sprinkled with chopped coriander.

5. Pour the sauce for dipping

SNACK: CURRIED CASHEWS

Makes 2 servings

Ingredients

- 3 cups cashews, whole or pieces
- 2 Tablespoons curry powder
- 2 Tablespoons water
- 1 Tablespoon honey
- 1 Teaspoon olive oil
- 1 Tablespoon sea salt, or add to taste

Directions

1.Preheat the oven to 250F and line a baking sheet with parchment paper.

2. Mix the ingredients and toss with the cashews.

3. Spread the nuts in an even layer and roast for 35-40 minutes.

4. Transfer to an airtight container.

5. Serve and enjoy!

DINNER: FISH & GRAPES SALAD
Makes 2 Servings

Ingredients

- 2 fish fillets
- ½ tbsp. coconut oil
- 1 large romaine lettuce - chopped
- 1/4 avocado - thinly sliced
- 2 stalks celery - finely chopped
- ½ red onion - finely chopped
- 1/3 cup extra virgin olive oil
- 1 tablespoon mustard
- 3 tablespoons fresh lemon juice
- 1 clove garlic - chopped or 1/8 tablespoon garlic powder
- Green olives
- Red grapes
- Salt and pepper

Directions

1. In a skillet, heat the coconut oil over medium heat.

2. Add fish and let it brown without overcooking on each side - about 2 minutes each side.

3. In a large bowl, combine the fish, lettuce, celery, red onion, avocado slices, olives and grapes.

4. In a separate bowl, whisk together olive oil, mustard, lemon juice, and garlic

5. Season to taste with salt and pepper.

6. Drizzle the salad with the dressing and mix well.

7. Serve immediately and enjoy!

WEEK 4

BREAKFAST OPTIONS

★ Omelet with Chanterelle mushroom & herbs

★ Energy Muesli

★ Chai Coco-Banana Smoothie

★ Tropical Smoothie

★ Potato Pesto Breakfast Skillet

★ Easy Paleo Scramble

★ Paleo smoothie

LUNCH OPTIONS

★ Colorful Salad

★ Wok Chicken & Broccoli

★ Red Cabbage Salad & Tuna

★ Greek Bean Salad

★ Ceviche shrimp

★ Chickpeas with chicken breasts

★ Paleo-styled Antipasto Salad

SNACK OPTIONS

★ Vanilla Pumpkin Seed Clusters

★ Paleo Appetizer with Fresh Figs

★ Paleo Avocado

★ Coconut Lemon Energy Balls

★ Paleo Baba-Ghanoush

★ Super Energetic Drink

★ nuts and dried fruits

DINNER OPTIONS

★ Stir Fried Beef with Vegetables

★ Beef Curry with Spinach and Potatoes

★ Carbonara Spaghetti

★ Creamy Lemon Chicken with Asparagus and Mushrooms

★ Thai Basil Beef Balls

★ Paleo Avocado Burgers with Caramelized Balsamic Onions

★ Pumpkin Gratin

DAY 1

BREAKFAST: OMELET WITH CHANTERELLE MUSHROOM & HERBS
Makes 2 Servings

Ingredients

- 4 eggs
- 2 large handfuls of chanterelles mushrooms
- 3 tbsp. olive oil for cooking
- 2 tbsp. tablespoons water
- Fresh herbs of your choice (parsley, rosemary, coriander) -chopped
- Sea salt

Directions

1. Rinse the mushrooms in clean water, and cut the stem.
2. In a medium saucepan, add 2 tablespoons of olive oil over low heat.
3. Stir in the mushroom in the olive oil at high heat and gradually decrease the heat.
4. Reduce to low heat and season with salt.
5. Remove the mushrooms from the pan and set aside in a bowl.

6. In a separate bowl, whisk 2 eggs and add a tablespoon of water.

7. Mix well until smooth.

8. In the cooking pot, heat a tablespoon of olive oil.

9. Pour the eggs and herbs into the pan, making sure to cover the entire surface.

10. Use a spatula to flip the omelet gently.

11. When your omelet is ready, fill one-half with 1/2 portion of mushrooms and close the other half of the omelet over

12. Allow to cook for 1 to 2 minutes.

13. Remove from heat and place the omelet onto a plate.

14. Add the other half remaining portion of chanterelles on the omelet with fresh herbs

15. Serve immediately and enjoy!

LUNCH: COLORFUL SALAD
Makes 4 Servings

Ingredients

- 1/2 purple cabbage
- 1/2 curly salad
- 1 yellow bell pepper
- 4 oranges tomatoes
- 10 Cherry tomatoes
- 8 Radish

- 1/2 Pineapple –sliced
- 1 handful Pumpkin seeds
- 4 tbsp. dressing of your choice

Directions

1. Clean, Peel, slice and chop all of the vegetables into desired cuts

2. Mix them in a bowl until well-combined

3. Sprinkle with pumpkin seeds and add your favorite dressing

4. Serve immediately and enjoy!

SNACK: VANILLA PUMPKIN SEED CLUSTERS
Makes 2 Servings

Ingredients

- 1/2 cup pumpkin seeds
- 2 tsp. honey
- 2 tsp. coconut sugar
- 1 tsp. vanilla extract
- Water (previously boiled)

Directions

1. Preheat oven to 300 F.

2. In a medium bowl, combine the honey, coconut sugar and vanilla.

3. Stir to create a thick paste then add a small drop of boiled water to thin it out for a smooth syrup

4. Pour in the pumpkin seeds and stir them around in the mixture to coat evenly.

5. Add a generous tsp. full of the pumpkin seeds onto a baking sheet

6. Repeat until it's all used up and cook for 15-20 minutes until most of the seeds have browned

7. Take out of the oven and leave to cool for a few minutes.

8. Once they've cooled a little you can press the clusters together to make sure they don't fall apart.

9. Serve and topping or as a cereal and enjoy!

DINNER: STIR FRIED BEEF WITH VEGETABLES
Makes 2 Servings

Ingredients

- 12 ounces of steak - cut into strips
- Broccoli and cauliflower florets
- Baby carrots (or vegetables of your choice)
- 1 white onion - thinly sliced
- 1 clove garlic - minced
- 1 tsp. ground ginger
- ½ cup water
- 2 tbsp. of coconut oil
- Salt and pepper

Directions

1 In a small bowl, combine water, ground ginger, and chopped garlic

2. Season with salt and pepper to taste.

3. Heat the coconut oil in a large skillet or wok over medium heat

4. Sauté beef until cooked through, about 4-6 minutes.

5. Remove the steak from the pan.

6. In the same pan, cook the onions, broccoli, cauliflower and carrots about 5 minutes.

7. Then, add the beef in the pan and add the mixture from the small bowl into the pan.

8. Let it cook for 2-3 minutes, then remove from heat.

DAY 2

BREAKFAST: ENERGY MUESLI
Makes 1 Serving

Ingredients

- 1 cup of coconut milk,
- 1/4 cup of oatmeal,
- 1/2 Banana (sliced)
- 1 tbsp. Peanut puree,
- 1 tsp. Raw Honey – organic
- 1 tsp. flaxseed oil

Directions

1. Put all ingredients in a bowl and mix the muesli.
2. Serve immediately and enjoy!

LUNCH: WOK CHICKEN & BROCCOLI
Makes 2 Servings

Ingredients

- 1 broccoli head
- 1 cup Chicken breast
- 1 Garlic clove
- 1 onion
- 1/2 cup Tamari
- 1 tsp. Olive oil
- Pepper

Directions

1. Cut the broccoli and steam for until softened.
2. Cut the onion into strips, fry in a pan with olive oil.
3. Press the garlic and add it to the pan
4. Cut the chicken into small pieces and sauté the onions and garlic.
5. Add broccoli to the skillet and the tamari sauce to mix
6. Season with pepper
7. Serve immediately and enjoy!

SNACK: PALEO APPETIZER WITH FRESH FIGS
Makes 4 Servings

Ingredients

- Bacon
- 4 fresh figs - cut lengthwise
- ¼ goat cheese - cut into small pieces
- 2 tbsp. Honey
- thyme

Directions

1. Preheat oven to 350 F
2. Fry the bacon in a frying pan and put them on a plate lined with paper towel
3. With the back of a spoon, gently press the flesh of figs to dig inside the fruit
4. In a bowl, combine the bacon, goat cheese, and honey
5. Add the mixture to the figs
6. Sprinkle the thyme on figs
7. Bake for 7 minutes
8. Serve immediately and enjoy!

DINNER: BEEF CURRY WITH SPINACH AND POTATOES
Makes 4 Servings

Ingredients

- 2 cups minced beef
- 2/3 cup spinach
- 1 tbsp. olive oil
- 2 cloves of garlic
- 2 tomatoes – chopped
- 4 potatoes - peeled and cut into 4 or 6
- 2cm turmeric root
- 1 tsp. curry powder
- Salt & pepper

Directions

1. Brown the ground beef for about 7 minutes on medium heat with olive oil
2. Add cloves of garlic tomatoes
3. Stir well constantly
4. While cooking the meat, peel and grate the turmeric root
5. Stir freshly grated turmeric, curry, salt and pepper into the meat mixture

6. Cook for 3 minutes.

7. Place them in the spiced minced meat mixture by pressing them a little.

8. Continue cooking, covered, for 10 minutes.

9. If necessary, add water.

10. Prick the potatoes to ensure softness.

11. Add the spinach leaves to the meat mixture.

12. Stir gently and quickly cook for 2 more minutes.

13. Serve immediately and enjoy!

DAY 3

BREAKFAST: CHAI COCO-BANANA SMOOTHIE

Makes 1 Serving

Ingredients

- 2 frozen bananas
- 2 tablespoons coconut milk
- 1/4 teaspoon of vanilla, cinnamon, cloves and ginger
- 1 cup of water

Directions

1. Place all ingredients into your blender
2. Blend until smooth.
3. Serve immediately and enjoy!

LUNCH: RED CABBAGE SALAD & TUNA
Makes 2 Servings

Ingredients

- Half of a big red cabbage
- 1 can of tuna
- 1 tbsp. sesame seeds
- 2 tbsp. pumpkin seeds
- Oil – hazelnut, walnut or olive
- Balsamic Vinegar
- Salt

Directions

1. With a grater, finely grate the red cabbage.
2. Crumble the tuna and mix in with the cabbage.
3. Season with balsamic vinegar, olive oil, salt, and lemon juice (optional).
4. Quickly toast the pumpkin seeds in a pan for 5 minutes
5. In each plate, sprinkle the cabbage salad spoon of pumpkin seeds and a hulled sesame spoon.
6. Serve immediately and enjoy!

SNACK: PALEO AVOCADO
Makes 2 Servings

Ingredients

- 1 avocado
- 1 lemon- freshly juiced
- 1 tbsp. onion - chopped
- 5 oz. wild tuna
- Sea salt and pepper to taste

Directions

1. Cut the avocado in half and scoop the middle of both avocado halves into a bowl - leaving a shell of avocado flesh about ¼-inch thick on each half.
2. Add lemon juice and onion to the avocado in the bowl and mash
3. Add tuna, salt, and pepper, and stir to combine.
4. Adjust flavor with sea salt and pepper, if needed.
5. Fill avocado shells with tuna salad
6. Serve immediately and enjoy!

DINNER: CARBONARA SPAGHETTI
Makes 2 Servings

Ingredients

- 1 large spaghetti squash
- 1 onion – chopped
- 2/3 cup Bacon
- 7 oz. coconut cream
- 3 Egg yolks
- Olive oil
- Salt and pepper

Directions

1. Preheat the oven to 350 F
2. Cut the squash in half lengthwise and remove the seeds.
3. Put the two halves in a bowl
4. Fill it halfway with hot water, then bake for 30 minutes.
5. Collect the pulpit of the squash with a fork – this will allow the "spaghetti" to form naturally
6. Peel and cut the onion and fry in a pan with a little olive oil.
7. Add the diced bacon and cook.

8. Add the cream and cook a little, then the egg yolks and mix well.

9. Add the spaghetti and mix.

10. Adjust seasoning to taste

11. Serve immediately and enjoy!

DAY 4

BREAKFAST: TROPICAL SMOOTHIE
Makes 1 Serving

Ingredients

- 1 cup papaya – ripened
- 2-3 Small guavas
- 1 sprig of parsley
- 1 tsp. lemon juice – freshly squeezed
- 1/2 tsp. ginger –chopped
- 1 tsp. flax seed
- 1 tsp. brown sugar, maple syrup, or stevia (optional)
- 3-4 ice cubes

Directions

1. Wash and clean all fruit

2, Once prepared, blend everything together with ice

3. Serve immediately and enjoy

LUNCH: GREEK BEAN SALAD
Makes 2 Servings

Ingredients

- 21 oz. of white beans - canned
- 8 dried tomatoes
- 10-ounce cherry tomatoes elongated,
- 7 oz. feta,
- 40 black olives,
- 1 red onion,
- 2 tbsp. olive oil,
- 4 tbsp. red balsamic vinegar.

Directions

1. Drain the beans and place them in a bowl.
2. Cut the dried tomatoes.
3. Wash and cut tomatoes into two the tomatoes.
4. Cut the feta into cubes.
5. Pit the olives and cut them into quarters
6. Peel the onion and cut it into slices.
7. Mix together and season with oil, vinegar and spices.
8. Serve immediately and enjoy!

SNACKS: COCONUT LEMON ENERGY BALLS
Makes 18 Servings

Ingredients

- dates, pitted & chopped
- 1 lemon, zest
- lemons, juice
- ¼ cup chia seeds
- 1.5 cup raw almonds
- ½ cup shredded coconut - unsweetened
- ¼ tsp. sea salt
- 1 tbsp. virgin coconut oil

Directions

1. Zest 1 lemon and set it aside.

2. Juice 2 lemons into a small bowl.

3. Add the chia and mix well.

4. Combine almonds and dates in the bowl of a large food processor.

5. Process until finely ground, about 60 seconds.

6. Add shredded coconut, sea salt, coconut oil, reserved zest, and chia/lemon juice mixture.

7. Process until the mixture is lumpy and moist, about 60 seconds.

8. Roll the mixture into 2" balls. Sprinkle with coconut, if desired.

9. Refrigerate 30 minutes to set.

10. Serve immediately and enjoy!

*Keep refrigerated in a sealed container.

DINNER: CREAMY LEMON CHICKEN WITH ASPARAGUS AND MUSHROOMS
Makes 4 Servings

Ingredients

- 3-4 large chicken breasts
- 8 asparagus spears - medium-sized cut into 1 inch pieces
- 8 oz. sliced mushrooms
- 2 tbsp. coconut oil
- 3 garlic cloves - crushed
- ¾ cup coconut milk –organic
- Juice of 1 lemon – freshly squeezed
- Zest of 1 lemon
- Salt, to taste

Directions

1. Begin by heating up a large skillet to medium-medium high heat.
2. Once hot, add 1 tbsp. coconut oil.
3. Place chicken in pan, heat about 3 minutes per side, and set aside
4. Add remaining coconut oil, if needed.
5. Toss in crushed garlic, asparagus, and mushrooms.
6. Sauté until asparagus is crispy, and mushrooms are soft and fragrant - about 10 minutes
7. Return the chicken to the pan.
8. Add in coconut milk, lemon juice, and lemon zest.
9. With the skillet over medium-high heat, and cover.
10. Wait until the mixture bubbles, then reduce medium-low heat.
11. Cook for an additional 3-5 minutes or until the chicken is cooked through.
12. Add salt to taste and serve with rice, pasta, or zoodles.
13. Serve immediately and enjoy!

DAY 5

BREAKFAST: POTATO PESTO BREAKFAST SKILLET
Makes 1 Serving

Ingredients

For the Pesto:
- 1 cup fresh basil
- 1 cup fresh kale
- 1/3 cup raw slivered almonds or regular almonds
- 2 large cloves garlic
- 2 tbsp. extra-virgin olive oil
- 1 tsp. lemon juice
- 1 tsp. fine pink sea salt
- 1/2 tsp. freshly ground pepper
- Optional: 1/4 tsp. red pepper flakes

For Everything Else:
- 1 tbsp. extra-virgin olive oil.
- 1 large Japanese sweet potato (or regular sweet potato), sliced thinly
- 2-4 purple potatoes, sliced thin
- 2 Eggs – organic

Directions

1. Heat oil in a skillet
2. Add in sliced potatoes and let cook for 5 minutes
3. Add in 1 tbsp. of water and cover skillet with a lid
4. After 5 minutes, remove lid and toss potatoes
5. While cooking a little while longer, toss pesto ingredients into your high-speed blender
6. Pour pesto over potatoes and toss until fully coated
7. Crack in eggs and let cook for 5-10 minutes
8. Once egg whites are cooked, remove from heat, and sprinkle with red pepper flakes
9. Serve immediately and enjoy!

Lunch: Ceviche shrimp
Makes 2 Servings

Ingredients

- 12 Pcs. Peeled Shrimp
- 1 Lemon
- 1 red onion
- 2 Peppers: 1 yellow, 1 red
- Parsley

Directions

1. Place the shrimp in a small dish and cover them with lemon juice.
2. Refrigerate for at least two hours.
3. Discard the lemon juice, dry the shrimp and mix with finely chopped onion and diced peppers.
4. Add chopped parsley and mix again.
5. Serve chilled and enjoy!

SNACK: PALEO BABA-GHANOUSH
Makes 2 Servings

Ingredients

- 2 large eggplants;
- 2 garlic cloves, minced
- 2 tbsp. fresh lemon juice
- 2 tsp. extra-virgin olive oil
- Salt and pepper to taste
- 2 tbsp. tahini (optional)
- 1 tsp. cumin (optional)
- Fresh parsley, for garnishing - optional

Directions

1. To roast the eggplants, either use your grill, the open flame of a gas stove or your oven to 400 F.

2. Put the roasted eggplants in a bowl of cold water then peel off the skin.

3. Place the roasted eggplant, garlic, lemon juice, tahini, olive oil, cumin in a blender

4. Blend until smooth.

5. Season to taste with salt and pepper.

6. Cool in the refrigerator and serve with olive oil on top and fresh parsley.

7. Serve immediately and enjoy!

DINNER: THAI BASIL BEEF BALLS
Makes 2 Servings

Ingredients

- 4 cloves garlic - minced
- 2 lbs. ground beef
- 1/2 cup almond flour
- 2 eggs
- 1 roasted red pepper - chopped
- 1/4 cup wheat-free soy sauce

- 1 tsp. fish sauce
- 1 tsp. Sriracha, chile or hot sauce
- 1 handful fresh basil leaves - chopped
- 1 lime, freshly zested
- Salt

Directions

1. Preheat oven to 400 F.
2. In a small skillet, heat up a teaspoon or 2 of your fat of choice
3. Sauté the garlic until it's golden.
4. In a large bowl, whisk together all ingredients except the beef.
5. Add the beef and mix well, making sure everything is well-combined.
6. Portion out the mixture, using a cookie scoop, onto a parchment or baking sheet.
7. Place baking sheet in the oven until cooked through and the top has slightly browned, about 20-30 minutes.
8. Serve immediately and enjoy!

DAY 6

BREAKFAST: EASY PALEO SCRAMBLE
Makes 2 Servings

Ingredients

- 8 oz. ground pork or breakfast sausage
- 1 cup shredded sweet potato or butternut squash
- 2 cup hearty greens
- 4 tomatoes - halved
- 2 eggs, beaten
- Sea salt & pepper, to taste

For toppings:

- chopped chives/scallions
- 1 avocado

Directions:

1. In a cast iron pan or nonstick skillet, cook the meat over medium heat until brown and crumbled.
2. Add the shredded carrot/squash and the greens and cook until wilted, about 3 minutes.
3. Add the cherry tomatoes and stir to warm them, about 30 seconds.
4. Turn the heat to medium-low and add the eggs.
5. Stir gently until eggs are just set.
6. Season with sea salt and pepper and top with garnishes, as desired.
7. Serve immediately and enjoy!

LUNCH: CHICKPEAS WITH CHICKEN BREASTS
Makes 2 Servings

Ingredients

- 10 oz. chickpeas - canned
- 2 chicken breasts
- 2 tsp. canola oil
- 1 large onion chopped
- 2 red peppers
- 1 zucchini
- 4 pickles
- 4 tbsp. white balsamic vinegar
- 1 cup of water
- 1 lemon
- 1 chili

Directions

1. Wash, clean and dry the chicken breasts and cut them into pieces.
2. Fry in canola oil, season and set aside.
3. Peel the onion and wash peppers.
4. Slice them and fry them in olive oil.
5. Cut the zucchini and add it with the peppers and onion.
6. Cut the cucumbers and put them to heat with other vegetables.
7. Put the chickpeas, vegetables and meat in a bowl.
8. Mix the vinegar, oil, water, lemon, and spices and pour over the salad.
9. Serve immediately and enjoy!

SNACKS: SUPER ENERGETIC DRINK
Makes 1 Serving

Ingredients

- 2 apples – organic
- 1/2 cup raspberries
- 1 lemon - freshly squeezed
- 1 tbsp. Raw Honey –organic
- 1 tsp. acerola powder
- 1 tbsp. chia seeds

Directions

1. Rinse apples and cut into 4 pieces

2. Rinse raspberries

3. Place both ingredients into the juicer

4. Squeeze the lemon juice and add to the fruit mixture

5. Add honey, acerola powder and mix

6. Top with chia seeds and pour into a bottle

7. Place in the fridge and let cool

8. Serve cold and enjoy!

DINNER: PALEO AVOCADO BURGERS WITH CARAMELIZED BALSAMIC ONIONS

Makes 6 Servings

Ingredients

- 1½ pounds of lean ground beef {makes six ¼lb. burgers}
- 1 teaspoon of salt
- 1 teaspoon of pepper
- 1 teaspoon of garlic powder
- 2 tablespoons of coconut oil
- 2 small onions - thinly sliced
- 2 tablespoons of balsamic vinegar
- 1 beef steak tomato -sliced into 6 thick slices
- 2 avocados - sliced

Directions

1. Heat a medium skillet over medium-high heat.
2. Add 1 tablespoon of coconut oil, once melted add in onions.
3. Sauté until caramelized, stir occasionally - About 10-15 minutes
4. Add in balsamic vinegar. Sauté for another 5 minutes, stir occasionally, then set aside.
5. Form six ¼lb. burgers with the lean ground beef.

6. Lightly season both sides with salt, pepper, and garlic powder.
7. Heat a large skillet over medium-high heat.
8. Add 1 tablespoon of coconut oil.
9. Place the burgers in the skillet and sauté each side for 3-5 minutes
10. Remove from skillet and let sit for 1 minute.
11. Assemble burgers and place 1 large slice of beef steak tomato on a plate, then the burger, then 2 tablespoons of the balsamic caramelized onions, and top with sliced avocado
12. Serve immediately and enjoy!

DAY 7

BREAKFAST: PALEO SMOOTHIE
Makes 1 Serving

Ingredients

- 1 beet - fresh
- 1 cup kale
- 1 mango - ripened
- 1 banana – ripened
- 1/2 cup pineapple - fresh
- 1 tbsp. chia seeds
- 1 can full-fat coconut milk – organic

Directions

1. Combine all ingredients in a blender and pulse until smooth results
2. Serve chilled and enjoy!

LUNCH: PALEO-STYLED ANTIPASTO SALAD
Makes 2-4 Servings

Ingredients

- 1 large head romaine lettuce - chopped
- 4 oz. prosciutto - cut in strips
- 4 oz. salami or pepperoni - cubed
- ½ cup artichoke hearts - sliced
- ½ cup olives,
- ½ cup hot or sweet peppers - pickled or roasted
- Italian Dressing, to taste

Directions

1. Combine all ingredients together and mix well
2. Serve immediately and enjoy!

SNACKS: NUTS AND DRIED FRUITS
Makes 2 Servings

Ingredients

- 2/3 cup mixed nuts (walnuts, cashews, hazelnuts, almonds, etc.)
- 1 cup of dates, figs or a mixture of both
- 1 tbsp. grated coconut - organic
- 3 tsp. coconut oil – extra-virgin

• raisins - optional

Directions

1. Place all ingredients in a food processor and blend until a dough in which it remains walnut pieces.
2. Pour the mixture into a bowl and add the sunflower seeds
3. Take a bit of dough to form a ball so it keeps its shape.
4. Place in the fridge for at least 1 hour.
5. Serve and enjoy!
*The balls can be stored in the fridge in an airtight container for several days

DINNER: PUMPKIN GRATIN
Makes 2-4 Servings

Ingredients

- 1 large pumpkin
- 1 cup minced beef
- 2 carrots
- 1 onion
- 1 shallot
- Coconut milk - organic
- Olive oil
- Salt and pepper

Directions

1. Preheat oven to 300 F.
2. Peel the pumpkin, remove the seeds and cut into medium size cubes.
3. Put them in a large pot of salted water and cook covered over medium heat.
4. When cooked, put the pumpkin in a blender for smooth and creamy mashed pumpkin.
5. Add coconut milk for creaminess.
6. Peel the carrot, onion and shallot.

7. Cut them into small slices and put in a pan with the olive oil over medium heat.

8. Cook for about 3 minutes.

9. Add the minced meat and do a little brown the meat on the fire

10. Mix all with the pumpkin, then pour into a baking dish.

11. Bake at 300 F for about 10 minutes.

CONCLUSION

The aim of the book was to explain the Paleo diet in detail and all its associated aspects. The Paleo diet is considered to be one of the best diets in the world and this has been proven throughout the years.

It is essential to understand that you aren't going to experience benefits right away. Just like everything in life, it requires hard word, dedication, and time. Most people begin experiencing results within thirty days but based on your health condition and other associated factors, you could experience results either sooner or later. It is essential that you also exercise throughout the diet and stay hydrated. These are both significant things that are going to help you gain even more health benefits.

The Paleo diet is an excellent diet as long as you will be committed to it. This is something that many people don't understand and struggle with in the beginning. As already mentioned in the book, following the diet is going to mean that you are going to dedicate yourself both mentally and physically. This includes choosing the food you eat and prepare it.

I am more than happy to have shared all this information with you and hope that you are going to find it beneficial. Good luck on your journey to better physical and mental health. The fact that you have read this book is an excellent sign that you are willing to take control of your life and change it for the better.

This is the start of a completely new and healthier life.

www.ingramcontent.com/pod-product-compliance
Lightning Source LLC
Chambersburg PA
CBHW071343280526
45787CB00001B/197